the

CHAKRA

DIRECTORY

Discover Your Chakras for

HEALING & BALANCE

the

CHAKRA

DIRECTORY

Discover Your Chakras for

HEALING & BALANCE

Vicki Howie

chartwell
books

Brimming with creative inspiration, how-to projects, and useful information to enrich your everyday life, Quarto Knows is a favorite destination for those pursuing their interests and passions. Visit our site and dig deeper with our books into your area of interest: Quarto Creates, Quarto Cooks, Quarto Homes, Quarto Lives, Quarto Drives, Quarto Explores, Quarto Gifts, or Quarto Kids.

This edition published in 2021 by Chartwell Books,
an imprint of The Quarto Group
142 West 36th Street, 4th Floor
New York, NY 10018 USA
T (212) 779-4972 F (212) 779-6058
www.QuartoKnows.com

Chartwell titles are also available at discount for retail, wholesale, promotional, and bulk purchase. For details, contact the Special Sales Manager by email at specialsales@quarto.com or by mail at The Quarto Group, Attn: Special Sales Manager, 100 Cummings Center Suite 265D, Beverly, MA 01915 USA

10 9 8 7 6 5 4 3 2 1

ISBN: 978-0-7858-3938-5

Library of Congress Control Number: 2020952765

Conceived, designed, and produced by
The Bright Press, an imprint of The Quarto Group.
The Old Brewery, 6 Blundell Street,
London N7 9BH, United Kingdom.
T (0)20 7700 6700
www.QuartoKnows.com

Design and layout by Clare Barber; Cover design by Emily Nazer
Illustrations by Joanna Kerr

Printed in China

This book provides general information. It should not be relied upon as recommending or promoting any specific diagnosis or method of treatment for a particular condition, and it is not intended as a substitute for medical advice or for direct diagnosis and treatment of a medical condition by a qualified physician. Readers who have questions about a particular condition, possible treatments for that condition, or possible reactions from the condition or its treatment should consult a physician.

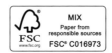

to the beautiful and resourceful editors,
lucy and stephanie, who helped me shape this book,
my beloved partner, Ross, who helped give it soul,
and you, dear reader, who inspired me to
write it. May you open all your chakras
and live life to the fullest!

CONTENTS

CHAPTER THREE

INTRODUCTION

As human beings, each and every one of us embodies an exquisite contradiction. We are simultaneously physical and spiritual. We are bound by time, and yet there is a part of us that is timeless. We experience worldly limitations, and still there is an aspect of us that is absolutely unlimited. If we want to experience our authentic wholeness, we need to bring these seemingly contradictory parts of ourselves into unity. The chakras are the bridge by which we do this and, in this book, you're going to learn what they are and how to work with them to unleash your highest potential.

THE RELUCTANT STUDENT

I wasn't always an enthusiastic chakra teacher and innovator. In fact, in the beginning, I was a very reluctant chakra student.

I was in love with yoga, so I signed up for teacher training. The chakras were a mandatory part of the curriculum, so I diligently learned their locations, qualities, and proper Sanskrit names in rote fashion. They didn't seem personally relevant to my life, but because I was a yoga teacher, they kept showing up in my work and my studies, until I knew a lot about them, without even trying.

Then, one day, when I had accumulated quite a bit of chakra understanding, I had a huge "Aha!" I suddenly realized that all my biggest issues were related to one chakra—the root.

In hindsight, it was obvious. For years I had been suffering from money issues; chronic fear and anxiety; and bowel, feet, and knee problems. I was changing

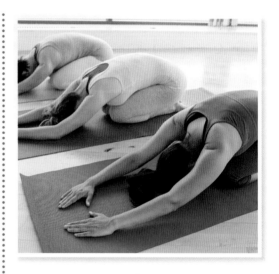

Yoga invites us to honor and utilize the seven powerful energy centers within us.

homes once or twice a year, and I had a visceral dislike for commitment, anything routine, and the color red. Add to that the fact that my father died suddenly when I was one year old (the most powerful root chakra development year) and my mom immediately turned to alcohol in order to cope. I was practically the poster child for a deficient first chakra.

A TURNING POINT

Diagnosing my main chakra weakness was a huge turning point for me. It gave me an actual place (the root) on which to focus my healing efforts. And that's exactly what I did!

I worked with stones and mantras and took up aromatherapy, yoga, and simple root chakra activities such as drumming, hiking, and communing with trees.

One day, I had a flash of insight that inspired me to get a root chakra tattoo and to create my Chakra Boosters Healing Tattoos™, and everything changed. My life shifted in countless positive, root-chakra-related ways. My chronic fear and anxiety disappeared, and I began waking up happy and inspired.

Now I am debt-free, joyously abundant, and have a deeply meaningful career that I love, where I get to work with the chakras and help people. And I'm living in my dream home in my favorite place on the planet—Sedona, Arizona.

YOUR JOURNEY

I share my story because I am in no way special or unique. You have these amazing energy centers in you. We all do! And as you learn to work with them in a skillful way, you will be able to create the shifts you desire and expand into your full potential. This book is going to show you the incredible chakra power that lies within you and how to fully utilize it.

In chapter one, you're going to learn all about your chakras. In chapter two, you'll discover how to assess the current state of your chakras, and, in the final chapter, you'll learn the best ways to heal and balance your chakras, and how to take your life to an entirely new level.

If you embrace this information with your whole heart, mind, and soul, there's nothing you can't do, be, or have. Let your chakra journey begin!

Wearing and using gemstones is one of the many ways you can heal your chakras.

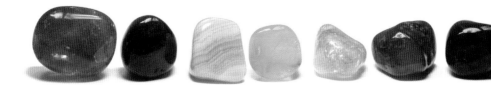

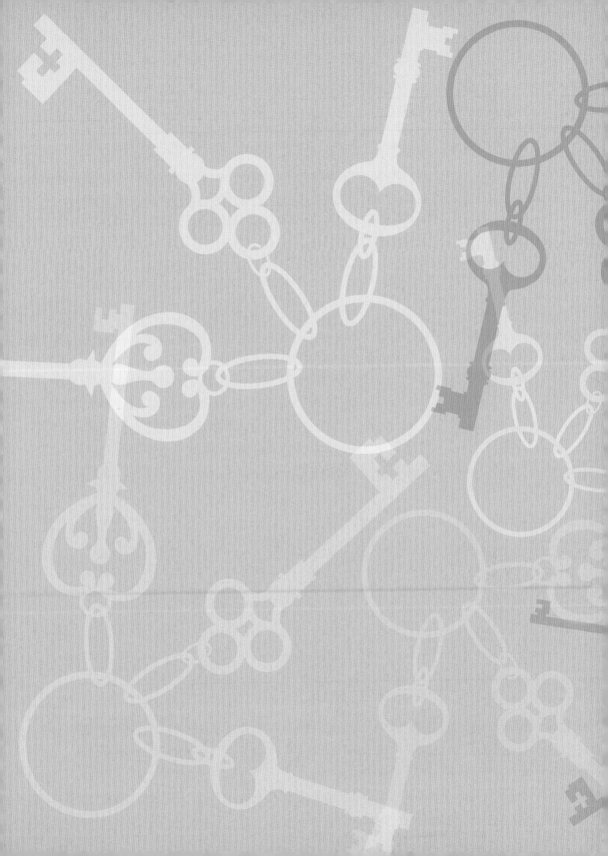

CHAPTER ONE

THE KEY to UNDERSTANDING YOUR CHAKRAS

O—➤ Discover the Seven Energy Centers that Hold Your Full Potential

O—➤ Explore Your Chakras with Engaging Exercises and Meditations

O—➤ Learn All About Your Aura and How to See and Feel It

O—➤ Find Out How Your Chakras Directly Affect Your Physical Body

WHAT ARE THE CHAKRAS?

Deep down each one of us knows that we are more than merely a body. We all feel our own essence—and the essence of others—underneath our physical forms. Quantum physics has shown quite clearly that matter is really just energy, which means that first and foremost you and I are vibrational beings.

The chakras are the key centers of your personal energy field that reside along your spinal column. They interface with your physical body through important nerve plexuses and glands, therefore they are the gateway through which your spirit affects your physical body.

SEVEN CHAKRAS

In the most popularly accepted system, there are seven chakras that span vertically from your tailbone to the top of your head. From the bottom up, they are: the root, sacral, solar plexus, heart, throat, brow, and crown.

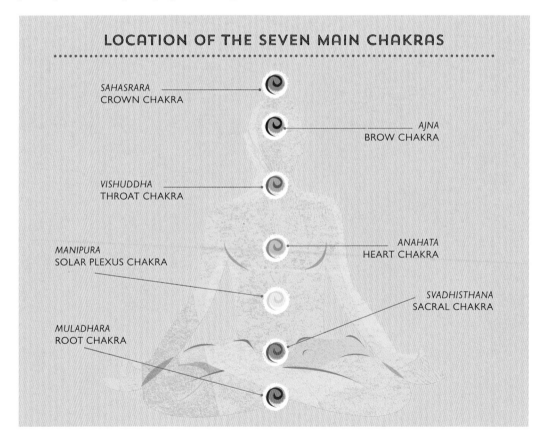

LOCATION OF THE SEVEN MAIN CHAKRAS

SAHASRARA
CROWN CHAKRA

AJNA
BROW CHAKRA

VISHUDDHA
THROAT CHAKRA

MANIPURA
SOLAR PLEXUS CHAKRA

ANAHATA
HEART CHAKRA

SVADHISTHANA
SACRAL CHAKRA

MULADHARA
ROOT CHAKRA

REVOLVING DOORS

The word "chakra" comes from the yoga-related language, Sanskrit, and it means "wheel" or "spinning disk." This is a pretty apt name for these energy centers, since each one spins like a mini-vortex. Still, it may serve you better to think of each chakra as a revolving door.

Just as revolving doors let people in and out, your chakras allow energy to move in and out of your body. They continually take energy in, assimilate it, and send it back out. In order for you to thrive, these doors must be healthy and open, and your energy flowing. When it is, you can live fully, taking in all that life has to offer and expressing all that you have to give.

your physical existence, while the more quickly vibrating upper chakras (five, six, and seven) relate to your spiritual experience. They are associated with your highest purpose—your psychic abilities, and your connection to the Divine, respectively.

The heart is the sweet balance point of your chakra field, the bridge between your physical and spiritual aspects. When your chakras are truly balanced and you are in your most energetically healthy state, you are naturally in a state of love.

Like revolving doors in a department store, your chakras are the bridge between your unseen inner world and the physical world outside of you.

ENERGETIC FREQUENCIES

Each chakra corresponds to a different energetic frequency, with the root being the densest and the crown the lightest. And each one relates to different aspects of your life—for example, wealth, power, sexuality, love, communication, psychic ability, and connection to the Divine.

The lower, more slowly vibrating chakras (one, two, and three) relate to

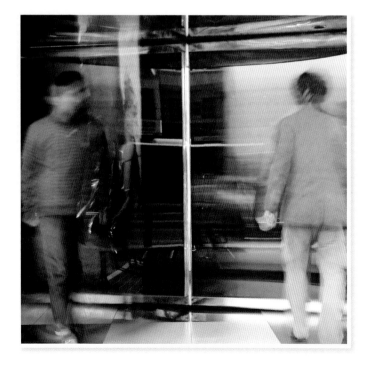

HOW THE CHAKRAS HAVE EVOLVED

The chakras were first discovered by devout Indian yoga practitioners between three thousand and four thousand years ago. The yogis of that era spent long hours meditating and exploring their inner worlds. From their practice, they were able to create maps of the human inner landscape, laying out the chakras and nadis (subtle energy pathways) in much the same way that early cartographers and explorers mapped the continents and seas of our planet.

Just as the earliest atlases of the world were not very accurate, because they relied on a lot of speculation, the earliest maps of our chakra system were merely first approximations. They were a good start, but they are not the gospel, despite coming from what many consider to be sacred texts. Our energy systems—and our understanding of them—have evolved and will continue to do so.

Every one of us can and should be a part of this evolution. As you read this book and do the exercises within it, feel into your own experience of your chakras. Question everything. Assume nothing. Own and name your own experience.

As I share a brief history of the chakras with you, be mindful of any tendency to consider ancient yogic texts as beyond reproach. The yogis who first discovered these systems were wise and dedicated men, but they weren't infallible, and our understanding of everything—including the chakras—evolves.

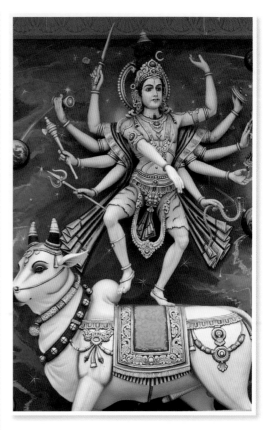

The Hindu god, Lord Shiva, dancing on a sacred cow.

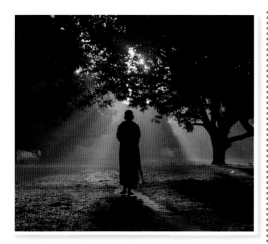

A Hindu monk walks at sunrise in Bangladesh.

THE CHAKRAS AND YOGA

The history of the chakras is inextricably tied to the history of yoga and the Hindu philosophies that evolved at the same time. The word "yoga" means "yoke" and stands for the yoking or unification of the individual self with the divine. The earliest yogis (meaning yoga practitioners) were passionately devoted to uniting the physical and spiritual aspects of themselves in order to experience the bliss of authentic wholeness.

The earliest-known writings about the chakras appear in the oldest yogic texts known to us, the *Vedas*, which were written sometime between 1500 and 500 BCE. It's generally accepted that the *Vedas* are a transcription of an even older oral tradition that was handed down by the Aryan people who invaded India in the second millennium BCE.

A second, very important, set of texts that laid out the chakras are the yoga *Upanishads*, written around 600 BCE. These texts are a collection of writings from proponents of slightly different schools of yogic thought, which explains why they contain some conflicting information. The most obvious variation is in the number of chakras attributed to the human body, with different *Upanishads* citing anywhere between five and eight.

KEYNOTE

Most English speakers pronounce the Sanskrit word chakra incorrectly. They use a "sh" sound at the beginning and an "ah" for the vowel sounds in the middle and at the end. This gives it a softer, sweeter tone, but if you want to stay true to the word's roots, the correct pronunciation uses the strong "ch" sound (as in church) at the beginning and "uh" (as in under) for the vowel sounds. Ultimately, how you pronounce the word chakra makes no difference to the way these potent energy centers affect your life, so choose the way that works best for you.

CHAKRAS IN THE WEST

Yoga and its energetic components, like the chakras, were largely unknown outside of India for thousands of years, and only really found their way into the Western psyche in the last century or so.

In the fall of 1918, a British man named Sir John Woodroffe (who wrote under the pen name of Arthur Avalon) published *The Serpent Power*, the first English-language book devoted to the chakras.

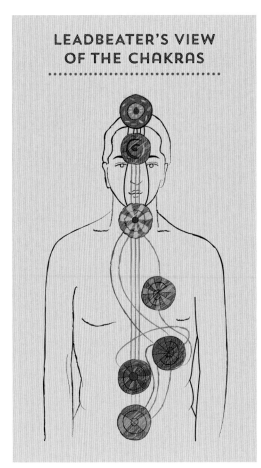

LEADBEATER'S VIEW OF THE CHAKRAS

Avalon's work took key elements of two very important Indian texts from the sixteenth century, the *Sat-Cakra-Nirupana* and the *Padaka-Pancaka*. He presented a six-chakra system and his book proved groundbreaking in that it gave people in the West a taste of India's deep understanding of the subtle systems of the human body.

Nearly a decade later, C. W. Leadbeater, a British theosophist and clairvoyant, added to Avalon's detailed and complex work when he published his book *The Chakras* in 1927. Leadbeater had the rare ability to actually see the chakras. and he described them in this way:

"The chakras or force-centres are points of connection at which energy flows from one vehicle or body of a man to another. Anyone who possesses a slight degree of clairvoyance may easily see them in the etheric double, where they show themselves as saucer-like depressions or vortices in its surface."

Leadbeater's book outlined a seven-chakra system, which is quite similar to the most widely embraced model in the world today. The only obvious differences are that he perceived the solar plexus and heart chakras as

♀ A diagram of Leadbeater's chakra
♂ system, which worked on a seven-chakra system similar to those used today.

More people are practicing yoga and becoming aware of their chakras than ever before.

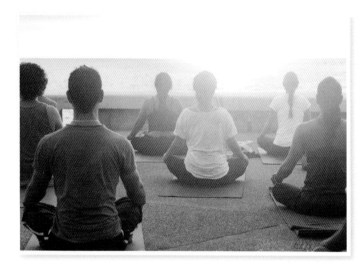

off-center, and his colors don't match the popular rainbow model most widely embraced today.

In the 1970s, when chakras were still relatively unknown in the US, a young American yoga practitioner and meditator, Anodea Judith, came onto the scene. After experiencing a couple of prophetic events regarding her chakras, Judith felt drawn to learn more about them and become a teacher. Since then, she has written numerous widely respected chakra books, including the classic *Wheels of Life* and, more recently, *Chakra Yoga*. Judith's writing has greatly influenced my understanding of the chakras with her more feminine, embodied approach. But perhaps the biggest influence of all has come from my talented yoga teachers and my own body. Through Anusara yoga, I learned how to be more grounded and access my chakras using precise Principles of Alignment. Coming to the mat became a practice of plugging into myself. I started to feel the subtle energy systems moving through me, and began to look and feel younger, better aligned, and more aware.

As yoga, meditation, and alternative healing practices grow at an unprecedented rate worldwide, I believe we are all contributing to the evolution of the chakras. Gone are the days where we need to turn to gurus for information about our own energy. We are the gurus. It's all within us, and increasing numbers of us are diving into the exploration with great reverence and determination.

These are exciting times. As a chakra student, I continue to explore the possibilities. And as a chakra innovator, I continue to create tools—like my Chakra Boosters Healing Tattoos™, my mantra-based music, and my Chakra Life Cycle System®—to further empower all of us energetically. I am delighted to be a part of our collective spiritual evolution, and I hope you are too!

YOU ARE A RAINBOW

At the start of my chakra studies, I was a reluctant student, because I didn't understand what these seven energy centers had to do with me. They seemed more abstract than actual. Then, one day I read that the colors of my chakras were the same as the colors of a rainbow. Wow. That blew me away! Why hadn't I realized that before?

I suddenly understood why I felt awe every time I saw a resplendent rainbow stretch across the sky. It was my own glorious potential writ large! My relationship with chakras got deeper that day, because the idea that I was a walking rainbow, full of possibility, felt real and inspiring to me. I hope it gives you the same feeling too, because you truly are a rainbow. Not sort of, but exactly. Your chakras are the same color spectrum as a rainbow.

NEWTON'S SPECTRUM

In the late 1600s, Sir Isaac Newton performed an experiment in which he beamed white light through a prism and got six distinct bands of color: red, orange, yellow, green, blue, and violet. He then sent those six colors back through a second prism, and again he got white light.

Newton's experiment is a perfect metaphor for the human chakra system. Our 3-D reality is like his prism. We come from pure white light, which is our spiritual essence. When we move into the physical world our essence gets refracted into a spectrum, revealing all the different colors within us, and eventually, when we die, we return to that pure white light again.

Interestingly, the seventh chakra, located just above the crown, is sometimes depicted as violet, and sometimes shown to be white. This is because it acts as a bridge between the highest point on our body, which is violet, and our pure spiritual essence, which is white.

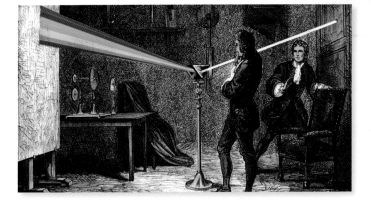

In 1665 Newton proved that white light contains the full color spectrum.

CHAKRA COLOR MEDITATION

1. Close your eyes and watch your breath, as you gently lengthen your inhales and exhales.

2. When you feel totally relaxed, imagine you're standing in front of a black-and-white cardboard cutout of your own body, and there is an empty circle where each chakra should be.

3. See yourself picking up a bright red crayon and boldly color in the area of your root chakra, at your tailbone. As you do this, feel how strong, stable, and safe your root chakra is.

4. Now, see yourself using a bright orange crayon to sensually color in your sacral chakra in the center of your pelvis. As you color it orange, feel how joyous, playful, and creative your sacral chakra is.

5. Pick up a bright yellow crayon and see yourself confidently color in your solar plexus chakra in your upper abdomen. As you color it yellow, feel the power and energy that radiates from your core.

6. Grab a glowing green crayon and gently color in your heart chakra in the center of your chest. As you color it green, feel how loving, compassionate, and healing your heart chakra is.

7. Use a bright blue crayon to color in your throat chakra. As you color it blue, feel how authentic, pure, and purposeful your throat chakra is.

8. Now imagine you have an indigo crayon, and color in your third-eye chakra—between your brows. As you color it indigo, feel how intuitive and wise your brow chakra is.

9. See yourself coloring in your crown chakra with a violet crayon, and as you color, see it turn white. Feel the immortality of your spiritual essence.

10. Now, using the white crayon, draw lines up and down your spinal channel, filling your body with infinite energy.

11. Allow this energy to continue to flow, and when you feel ready, gently open your eyes.

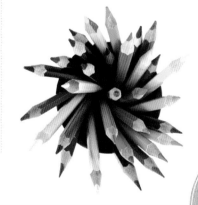

YOUR SEVEN CHAKRAS EQUAL 6+1

Although we talk about seven chakras, it's best to think of your chakras as a system of 6+1, because six of them reside within the physical field of your body, and one does not.

THE CROWN STANDS ALONE

Your crown chakra is unique: it resides off the body, and is directly connected to the Divine. This means that your highest chakra has only one upward vortex to Source energy. All the other chakras have both front and back vortices that can be measured for healing purposes.

In the chakra exploration exercise, you will get to feel the front vortex of each chakra. Pay close attention to the crown and you'll feel that it has no front or back vortex, because it doesn't operate like the six embodied chakras that are split into the duality of our physical world. In our 3-D experience, we have three dimensions of duality—up–down, left–right, and front–back.

Once you have tried the chakra exploration exercise, we will take a look at the qualities of each chakra such as its color, location, element, bodily sense, and more.

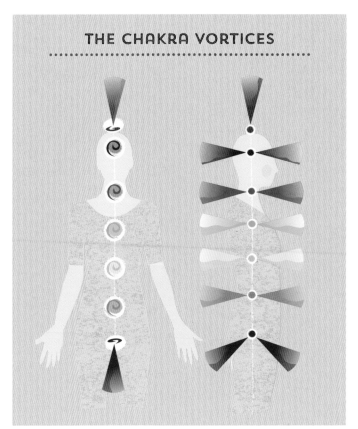

THE CHAKRA VORTICES

♀ The six embodied chakras all have a front and back portal, but the crown, which is connected to the Divine, does not. It only radiates to, and receives from, the upward spiritual portal, as you can see in this diagram of the vortices.

CHAKRA EXPLORATION

In this simple chakra exercise, you're going to explore the feeling of the subtle energy extending from each chakra.

1. Lie down on your back.

2. Rub your hands together then clap a few times to get them activated.

3. Close your eyes to become more kinesthetically aware, and place your right hand above the area of your root chakra at the lowest part of your groin. Start with your hand about one foot away from the body and very slowly begin to move it closer until you feel some cushiony energy coming from your body. For some people it feels a little energetically charged like tiny prickles, and for others, it's just soft and spongy. Feel into it and get curious.

4. Ask yourself questions like:
   • How far away from my body do I begin to feel my chakra energy?
   • What are its qualities?
   • Is the energy spongy, prickly, warm, or something else entirely?

5. Repeat this process for each chakra at the following locations:
   SACRAL CHAKRA—over the pelvis
   SOLAR PLEXUS CHAKRA—over the solar plexus (just below where the ribs begin to part)
   HEART CHAKRA—in the center of the chest
   THROAT CHAKRA—in the center of the throat
   BROW CHAKRA—in the center of the forehead, above and between the brows
   CROWN CHAKRA—just above the center of the head

6. If you wish, you can repeat the process again with your left hand to see if it feels different from the right. Make sure you clap and rub your hands a few times before repeating the process.

KEY CHAKRA TERMS

I'll be introducing some terms with which you may not be familiar, so let's define them:
• A **seed sound** is a short, sacred sound that helps to balance a chakra
• A **chakra need** is a basic developmental need that arises in each chakra in early childhood
• A **chakra right** is the inalienable, spiritual right that a chakra gives you (rights are verbs like "to be," "to feel," "to do," and so on).

THE ROOT CHAKRA

Your root chakra is located at the base of your spine and it's associated with the element of earth and your sense of smell. It governs your feet, legs, perineum, and rectum, and relates to your most basic, animalistic nature and your need to survive. It's red, which means it's heavier and denser than the other chakras, and it vibrates the most slowly.

The Sanskrit name for the root chakra is muladhara, which means "root support." This is the base chakra that connects you to Mother Earth and gives you a strong, stable foundation on which to build the rest of your life. It's also quite literally related to your roots in that it ties you to your natal family and your ancestors.

The root is the first chakra to develop, and it does so from birth to age seven. Before we come into this physical realm, we are pure consciousness. After conception, the root chakra starts connecting us to the Earth and our natal family so we can learn how to live in a body, be part of a tribe, and survive.

Your first chakra is about physical embodiment, so it's related to your overall health and vitality, as well as your ability to manifest physical things like money, good health, and other things you may desire. It's associated with simplicity, organization, and anything foundational in your life, as well as gravity and grounding, or what the yogis call *apana*, meaning "downward-moving energy."

Your root chakra directly influences your finances, work, family, and home life. It's also connected to your sense of safety and security, and your feeling of belonging in your body, with your tribe, and on this planet.

TAPPING INTO YOUR ROOT ENERGY

Close your eyes and imagine you are a very old, giant redwood tree. Feel how tall and sturdy you are and draw your focus to your deep, wide roots. Notice how they spread wide and anchor you into the Earth. Imagine them soaking in all the vital, robust nutrients you need, giving you vitality, strength, and stability. Feel into your roots for ten deep breaths, and, when you're ready, gently open your eyes.

ROOT CHAKRA QUALITIES

Color: Red
Sanskrit Name: Muladhara
Meaning: Root support
Location: Tailbone
Areas Affected: Perineum, rectum, legs, feet
Element: Earth
Sense: Smell
Gland: Testes (no root gland for women)

Seed Sound: Lam
Food Type: Meats and proteins
Stones: Garnet, ruby, black tourmaline, hematite, red jasper, bloodstone
Essential Oils: Sandalwood, patchouli, cedarwood, black spruce, vetiver
Celestial Body: Saturn
Main Focus: Physical existence
Basic Need: Certainty
Basic Right: To be
Positive Qualities: Stability, security, vitality, loyalty, prosperity, patience, tenacity, career success
Underactive Signs: Anxious, accident prone, financially unstable, constantly moving homes, disorganized, anorexic, chronic constipation, issues with knees, feet, bowels, blood, or bones
Overactive Signs: Inertia, addictions, hoarding, obesity, greed, depression, laziness, over-eating, issues with knees, feet, bowels, blood, or bones
Best Healing Methods: Aromatherapy, Hatha yoga, reflexology, gemstones, drumming, and didgeridoo

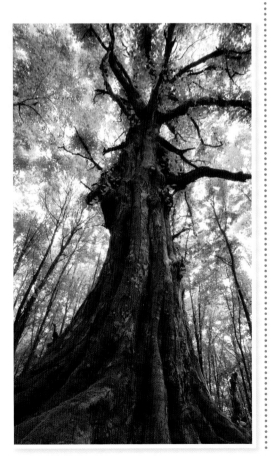

Trees, with their earthy energy and deep roots, are the perfect symbol of root chakra energy.

THE SACRAL CHAKRA

Your sacral chakra is located in the center of your pelvis and is associated with the element of water and your sense of taste. It's orange and it governs the area from your pelvic bowl up to your navel, including all your reproductive organs.

The second chakra is basically the opposite of the root chakra. Where the root chakra is about stability, stillness, and planning, the sacral chakra is about change, flow, and spontaneity. And whereas the root chakra is about learning to be in relationship with yourself, the sacral chakra is about learning to be in relationship with another.

It develops between the ages of 8 and 14, a period of great hormonal change and sexual awakening. During this time, we first pair off with a best friend, and a little later we begin to experiment with our first romantic crushes or couplings.

The sacral chakra is about intimacy, play, sexuality, creativity, emotions, and surrender. It may seem like a contradiction that a single chakra is simultaneously related to our sexuality and our childlike sense of fun and wonder, but those who engage in sacred sexual practices know that love-making can be very joyous and playful.

The Sanskrit name for this chakra is svadisthana, which means "one's own place," a perfect name for this highly personal, genitally oriented chakra.

Because the sacral chakra is the seat of our Divine feminine, all of us, men and women alike, create from our hips. This is the place from where we birth our curiosity, joy, and desire to deeply bond with another. And for women, of course, it's the chakra from which we literally give birth.

TAPPING INTO YOUR SACRAL ENERGY

Close your eyes and imagine you are a slow-moving river of molten lava making its way down the side of a volcano. Feel how warm, orange, and glowing you are as you sensually snake your way down through the cool, rocky terrain. Experience the easy way you glide around any barriers and continue on your way. Feel into your juicy, flowing sacral energy for ten deep breaths and, when you're ready, gently open your eyes.

SACRAL CHAKRA QUALITIES

Color: Orange

Sanskrit Name: Svadisthana

Meaning: One's own place

Location: Center of pelvis

Areas Affected: Genitals, reproductive organs, hips, lower back

Element: Water

Sense: Taste

Gland: Ovaries (no sacral gland for men)

Seed Sound: Vam

Food Type: Liquids

Stones: Carnelian, moonstone, coral, fire opal, orange calcite, amber

Essential Oils: Jasmine, orange blossom, fennel, rose, sage, ylang ylang

Celestial Body: Moon

Main Focus: Intimacy and emotions

Basic Need: Variety

Basic Right: To feel

Positive Qualities: Creativity, wide emotional range, joy, sexuality, fertility, pleasure

Underactive Signs: Sexual rigidity, fertility issues, genital problems, hip or sacroilliac joint problems, dehydration, resistance to change

Overactive Signs: Sexual promiscuity, codependence, lack of emotional control, bladder problems, STDs

Best Healing Methods: Water watsu, sacred sex, emotional release techniques, hip-opening yoga poses, massages, juice fasts

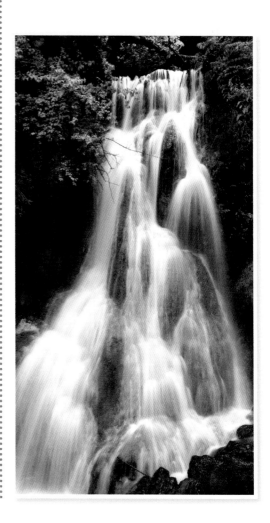

The sacral chakra is all about water, movement, and flow.

THE SOLAR PLEXUS CHAKRA

Your solar plexus chakra is located in the center of your torso above your navel, just below where your ribs part. It's yellow and it governs your midsection and all your digestive organs. It's also associated with the fire element and your sense of sight. The core chakra relates to your confidence, motivation, personal power, ego, and identity.

Many people don't know that the solar plexus chakra is also the home of our decision-making mind. It's where we create our worldly opinions and judgments, which explains why so many people say they have a "gut feeling" about something. And it's also why science has shown we have brain cells in our bellies!

The Sanskrit name for this chakra is manipura, which means "lustrous gem," because this is the place from which you shine. Your solar plexus is the energy center from which your value and true self-worth radiate. Not surprisingly, this chakra is also tied to fame.

Your core chakra develops from age 15 to 21, which explains why teens are so feisty and contrary. During these seven years, they are burning with a fiery passion to forge their own identity and independence.

The fire element in this chakra gives our body the energy needed to digest both food and ideas, and it also gives us the motivation, direction, and confidence to get things done.

Your solar plexus chakra is the seat of your will and personal power, so if it's strong, you feel in control of your destiny and if it's weak, you may feel like a victim in your own life.

TAPPING INTO YOUR SOLAR PLEXUS ENERGY

Close your eyes and imagine you are the Sun, burning bright and strong, radiating heat and light from your center. Feel into your awesome power and the brilliant way you shine. You are Source energy. You heat things up and make everything grow. You shine light everywhere you go. Experience your full solar magnificence for ten deep breaths and, when you're ready, gently open your eyes.

SOLAR PLEXUS CHAKRA QUALITIES

Color: Yellow

Sanskrit Name: Manipura

Meaning: Lustrous gem

Location: Solar plexus

Areas Affected: Stomach, liver, gallbladder, pancreas

Element: Fire

Sense: Sight

Gland: Adrenals (and pancreas)

Seed Sound: Ram

Food Type: Carbohydrates

Stones: Citrine, topaz, tiger's eye, fire agate, yellow apatite, golden calcite

Essential Oils: Lemon, peppermint, ginger, black pepper, cardamom, myrrh, pine, sage

Celestial Bodies: Sun, Mars

Main Focus: Personal power and identity

Basic Need: Significance

Basic Right: To act

Positive Qualities: Power, energy, confidence, charisma, will, motivation, mental clarity, levity

Underactive Signs: Digestion issues, kidney or liver problems, diabetes, timidity, chronic fatigue, constant confusion or indecision, low self-esteem, collapsed chest posture

Overactive Signs: Bullying, rage, ulcers, cancer of any digestive organs, hurrying

Best Healing Methods: Core-strengthening yoga or exercises, puzzles, sunbathing, yantra gazing, taking courageous action, fire-walking, TPQs

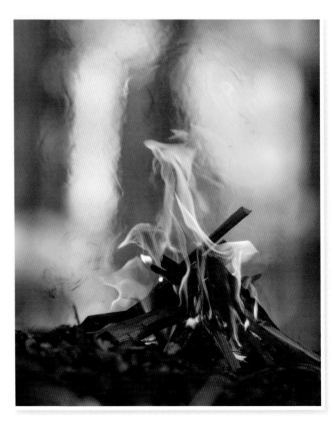

The solar plexus chakra is related to the element of fire and its transformational power.

THE HEART CHAKRA

Your heart chakra is located in the center of your chest, and it governs your heart, lungs, and diaphragm, as well as your arms and hands. It's green and is associated with the air element and your sense of touch. Not surprisingly, your heart chakra relates to compassion, gratitude, forgiveness, healing, and love.

Within your seven-chakra system, the heart, which develops the most from age 22 to 28, is the centerpiece. With three physically oriented chakras below it, and three spiritually oriented chakras above, it's a balancing point and a bridge that links body and mind, lust and reason, the earthly and the divine.

Its Sanskrit name is anahata, which is usually interpreted as "unstruck," but is also defined as "unbeaten" and "unwounded." The heart chakra is the pure innocent place of balance within us that cannot be hurt, even though our egoic selves often think it can.

The heart chakra is the center through which we heal. Its energy can move through our arms and hands to impart healing to others physically when we give massages or hugs, or energetically, when we do reiki or similar types of healing.

Because its element is air, which is related to thinking, the heart has a mind of its own, which is quite different from that of the third chakra. Whereas the solar plexus chakra likes to focus on the differences between things and judge and compare them, the heart chakra likes to accept and equalize. It sees the commonalities and connections.

When the heart chakra is healthy and balanced, it most closely resembles the conscious, loving energy of the Divine, and helps us to have thriving, loving relationships.

TAPPING INTO YOUR HEART ENERGY

Close your eyes and imagine you are a resplendent, spring meadow. People come from far and wide to rest their weary bodies on your vibrant, green grass, smell your fragrant flowers, and breathe in the vital oxygen of your life-giving trees. The peace of your pastures makes everyone feel healed and loved. Experience your sweet heart energy for ten deep breaths and, when you're ready, gently open your eyes.

HEART CHAKRA QUALITIES

Color: Heart
Sanskrit Name: Anahata
Meaning: Unstruck
Location: Center of chest
Areas Affected: From ribcage to shoulders (including heart, lungs, and diaphragm), arms, hands
Element: Air
Sense: Touch
Gland: Thymus (and heart)
Seed Sound: Yam
Food Type: Vegetables
Stones: Emerald, rose quartz, jade, pink tourmaline, malachite, moldavite
Essential Oils: Eucalyptus, rosemary, tea tree, thyme, cypress, ylang ylang, ginger
Celestial Body: Venus

Main Focus: Love and connection
Basic Need: To love and connect
Basic Right: To love and be loved
Positive Qualities: Love, trust, gratitude, forgiveness, compassion, kindness, healing, equanimity
Underactive Signs: Heart or breathing issues like asthma, sleep apnea, immune disorders, underactive thymus, emphysema, colds or pneumonia, lonely or antisocial
Overactive Signs: Always putting others first, people pleaser, breast or lung cancer, allergies
Best Healing Methods: Hugs, Emotional Freedom Technique, breath work, Ho'Oponopono, Reiki

Loving, hugging, and connecting with others opens your heart chakra.

KEYNOTE

There are only four true elements and they deal with the physical plane: earth, water, fire, and air. Once you get into the upper chakras, the "elements" are actually frequencies, of which there are three: sound (throat chakra), light (brow chakra), and pure consciousness (crown chakra).

THE THROAT CHAKRA

Your throat chakra is located in the center of your throat, and it governs the region from the base of your neck up to your ears. The jaw hinge is a key fifth chakra joint, as it often gets "locked" or causes issues when your throat center is out of balance.

This chakra is blue and is related to sound and your sense of hearing. This is important to note, because the throat center is often equated solely with expression. And, while communication in all its different forms—like talking, singing, and writing—is absolutely essential to our well-being, it's meaningless without the mature, spiritual ability to listen intently.

The Sanskrit name for the throat chakra is visuddha, meaning "purity." As the first of your more spiritually oriented upper chakras, it's challenging you to be more conscious with your communication.

Think of your throat chakra as a sort of filter and lie detector, because it only opens in a healthy way when you're authentic and honest, and it weakens when you tell lies, stifle your truth, keep toxic secrets, or try to be someone you're not.

The throat chakra is intrinsically connected to your true-life purpose, because when you're authentic and refuse to wear false masks or compromise, your highest destiny naturally emerges from everything you do. This energy center develops the most from age 29 to 35, a time when we all feel a need to mature and discover our real reason for being here.

A powerful throat chakra gives rise to authentic leadership. The great spiritual leaders of our time, Mahatma Gandhi and Martin Luther King, Jr., for example, were phenomenal communicators.

TAPPING INTO YOUR THROAT ENERGY

Close your eyes and imagine that you are the harmonious vibration of a glorious symphony. Your myriad instruments express complementary sounds, dancing together in joyous creation. Feel how you touch and inspire people with your inspiring concerto, from the lowest notes of your cello to the highest highs of your piccolo. Listen to the music of ten deep breaths and, when you're ready, gently open your eyes.

THROAT CHAKRA QUALITIES

Color: Blue

Sanskrit Name: Vishuddha

Meaning: Purity

Location: Center of throat

Areas Affected: Neck, jaws, mouth, ears

Element: Sound

Sense: Hearing

Gland: Thyroid

Seed Sound: Ham

Food Type: Fruits

Stones: Turquoise, lapis lazuli, sodalite, blue kyanite, blue calcite, aquamarine

Essential Oils: Clove, tea tree, blue chamomile, hyssop, eucalyptus

Celestial Body: Mercury

Main Focus: Authentic expression and life purpose

Basic Need: To grow spiritually and contribute

Basic Right: To express

Positive Qualities: Authentic, honest, purposeful, expressive, master artist, serves others, strong voice, great communicator

Underactive Signs: Hypothyroidism (underactive thyroid), TMJ (jaw disorder), sore throats, rarely speaks, quiet voice, pathological liar

Overactive Signs: Hyperthyroidism (overactive thyroid), tonsilitis, grinds teeth, talks too much, is too loud, poor listener

Best Healing Methods: Chanting mantras, crystal bowls, thyroid-stimulating yoga poses like Shoulder stand or Plow, and Fish, wear turquoise or lapis lazuli necklace

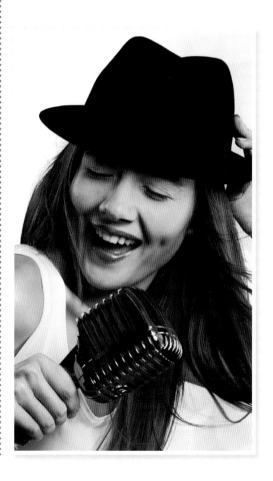

A strong throat chakra compels you to express your authentic voice.

THE BROW CHAKRA

Your brow chakra is located above and between the eyebrows and it governs the area from the sinuses up to the top of the head. The color of this center is indigo (deep purple-blue), and it's related to light and your sixth sense.

Many people prefer to call this center the "third eye," which is a very fitting name, because it gives you expanded vision and a wise, balanced perception, both inwardly and outwardly.

Its Sanskrit name is ajna, which means "command" and also "to perceive." Since the brow is the last of your embodied chakras, it is the highest, wisest point from which you can view things. You may wish to think of it as your command center or highest mind, and check in with it for all your key decisions.

This chakra naturally expands between the ages of 36 and 42, a period in which we typically find that our outer world accomplishments do not give our life enough meaning, so we turn inward, to the galaxy of possibility within us.

The third eye is the only spot on your body where your perceptions of duality dissolve. This is because the feminine and masculine energy channels of your spine—the ida and pingala (see page 42)—merge and become one here. This causes the two hemispheres of your brain to synchronize and work as one and allows you to better see patterns and decipher the bigger picture.

Because this chakra is connected to your dream states, it's associated with the pineal gland and not the pituitary, as some say. It's the home of your inner knowing, intuition, imagination and Higher Self.

TAPPING INTO YOUR THIRD-EYE ENERGY

Close your eyes and imagine that you are the original light that shines through everything. You are the twinkly, magical illumination of the stars and the warm slice of day that greets the dawn. You are far softer and more mythically powerful than the Sun, because you have the gift of insight. Feel into your warm, wise inner light for ten full breaths and, when you're ready, gently open your eyes.

BROW CHAKRA QUALITIES

Color: Indigo
Sanskrit Name: Ajna
Meaning: Command
Location: Behind center of forehead
Areas Affected: Sinuses, eyes, brain
Element: Light
Sense: Sixth (ESP)
Gland: Pineal
Seed Sound: Om
Food Type: Beauty (visual feast), and mind-altering substances
Stones: Azurite, labradorite, indigo kyanite, barite, blue iolite, purple charoite
Essential Oils: Clary sage, juniper, melissa, palmarosa, frankincense
Celestial Body: Neptune
Main Focus: ESP and clear perception
Basic Need: To connect with your Higher Self
Right: To perceive

Positive Qualities: Intuitive, insightful, equanimous, wise, perceptive, psychic, visionary, fair
Underactive Signs: Can't recall dreams, lacks intuition and self-trust, eye problems, sinus issues, overly prone to altitude sickness
Overactive Signs: Nightmares, hallucinations, bipolar, migraines, dyslexia, eye or sinus problems, insomnia, dizziness
Best Healing Methods: Meditation, intuitive exercises, making vision boards, lucid dreaming exercises

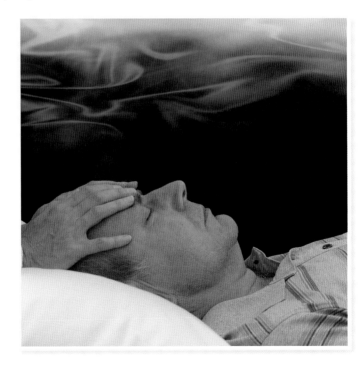

The brow chakra, also known as the third eye, relates to your psychic gifts and dream world.

THE CROWN CHAKRA

The crown chakra is different from the others in that it's not embodied and therefore not subject to the duality of our material world. It's related to pure consciousness, so it doesn't have many of the qualities of the other chakras. It isn't tied to any element, physical sense, seed sound, or food. It's beyond all of those. Instead, it relates to silence, stillness, and abstinence.

Strictly speaking, the crown chakra is violet. But as it expands upward into pure, unlimited source energy, it turns white, the indisputable hue of spirit. This seems fitting, since, as Newton proved, white is the color that contains every possible color of light, and spirit is the energy that contains all other energies.

Your crown chakra naturally expands between the ages of 42 and 49, a time when most of us are seeking a higher meaning for our life, and caring much less about mundane things.

Yogis have endeavored to fully open this highest chakra for centuries through meditation. They say that when you reach a deep state of one-pointed concentration that utterly stills the mind, your crown chakra opens and you experience enlightenment, a mystical state of knowing the underlying oneness of everything.

The Sanskrit name for this chakra is sahasrara, which means "thousand-fold," a metaphorical description of the many-petaled lotus that resides at the crown. Given that none of the other six chakras has more than 16 petals, it's clear that the crown is an auspicious chakra in a league of its own. This is likely due to the fact that it's seen as a gateway to the Divine, and a constant reminder of our true, spiritual nature.

TAPPING INTO YOUR CROWN ENERGY

Close your eyes and imagine you are a matrix of energy that spreads across the universe, through all galaxies, known and unknown, now and always. You are pure consciousness, the web that unifies everything, the awareness that lives beyond time and space. You are the brightest white light and the darkest black hole. Take ten deep breaths for everything in existence and, when you're ready, gently open your eyes.

CROWN CHAKRA QUALITIES

Color: Violet (to White)
Sanskrit Name: Sahasrara
Meaning: Thousand-fold
Location: Just above center of head
Areas Affected: Entire energy body
Element: None
Sense: None
Gland: Pituitary (and hypothalamus)
Seed Sound: Silence
Food Type: None (fasting)
Stones: Amethyst, Clear quartz, opal, violet sapphire, white calcite, diamond
Essential Oils: Lavender, rose, frankincense, helichrysum
Celestial Body: Jupiter
Main Focus: Oneness with everything

Basic Need: To connect with divinity
Basic Right: To know your true divine essence
Positive Qualities: Awareness, unity consciousness, understanding, wisdom, grace, bliss
Underactive Signs: Depression, apathy, extreme skepticism, Parkinson's, MS, OCD
Overactive Signs: God Complex, over-intellectualism, mental illness, stroke, Alzheimer's, insomnia, schizophrenia
Best Healing Methods: Prayer, meditation, fasting

The lotus flower that rises from the mud to the surface of the water is an iconic symbol of crown chakra energy.

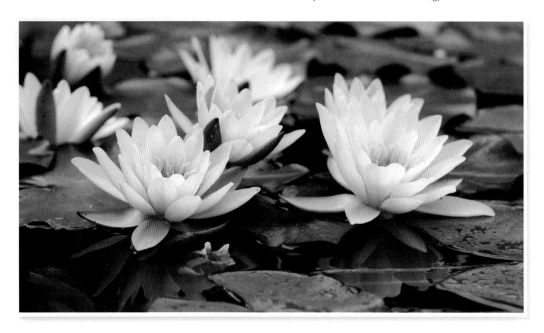

CHAKRA QUALITIES	1ST CHAKRA (masculine)	2ND CHAKRA (feminine)	3RD CHAKRA (masculine)
Color	Red	Orange	Yellow
Sanskrit name	Muladhara	Svadhisthana	Manipura
Meaning	Root support	One's own place	Lustrous gem
Location	Perineum/base of tailbone	Pelvis/sacrum	Solar plexus
Element	Earth	Water	Fire
Sense	Smell	Taste	Sight
Seed sound	Lam	Vam	Ram
Food type	Protein, meats	Liquids	Carbohydrates
Stones	Garnet Hematite Black tourmaline	Coral Carnelian Moonstone	Topaz Citrine Tiger's eye
Essential oils	Vetiver Patchouli Sandalwood	Jasmine Ylang ylang Orange blossom	Ginger Cardamom Peppermint
Main focus	Physical existence	Emotions and intimacy	Power and identity
Right	To have	To feel	To act
Basic need	Safety	Variety	Significance
Positive qualities	Stability Vitality Loyalty Prosperity Patience Tenacity Career success	Joy Creativity Adaptability Sensuality Fertility Emotional range Sexuality	Power Confidence Charisma Strong will Motivation Leadership Mental clarity
Malfunction (Over- or Underactive)	Bowel, blood or bone disorders, obesity, anorexia, anxiety, spaciness, chronic fear, materialism, addictions, skin problems, male infertility	Genital, sexual, and bladder issues, infertility, rigidity, hip or sacroiliac problems, dehydration, fear of intimacy	Digestion issues, kidney or liver problems, food allergies, rage, timidity, diabetes, ulcers, chronic fatigue, narcissism, low self-esteem

4TH CHAKRA (feminine)	5TH CHAKRA (masculine)	6TH CHAKRA (feminine)	7TH CHAKRA (unified)
Green	Blue	Indigo	Violet
Anahata	Visuddha	Ajna	Sahasrara
Unstruck	Purity	Command	1,000-petaled
Center of chest	Throat	Forehead center	Crown
Air	Sound	Light	Consciousness
Touch	Hearing	Intuition/ESP ("sixth sense")	None (beyond senses)
Yam	Ham	Om	Silence
Vegetables	Fruits	Beauty (visual feast)	Fasting
Jade Emerald Rose quartz	Sodalite Celestite Turquoise	Opal Azurite Lapis lazuli	Diamond Amethyst Clear quartz
Rosemary Thyme Eucalyptus	Clove Tea tree Blue chamomile	Clary sage Juniper Melissa	Helichrysum Lavender Frankincense
Love and connection	Self-expression and life purpose	Clear perspective and psychic abilities	Connection to spirit and wisdom
To love and be loved	To express	To perceive	To know
Love and be loved	Express truth	Connect with higher self	Oneness with the Divine
Love Trust Healing Gratitude Compassion Connection Forgiveness	Truth Purpose Expression Artistry Service Synchronicity Communication	Vision Intuition Dreams Insight Perception Equanimity Psychic abilities	Unity Wisdom Awareness Intelligence Understanding Miracles Bliss
Asthma, apnea heart or lung problems, breast cancer, allergies, immune disorders, loneliness, antisocial behaviors, thymus issues	Thyroid or hearing problems, teeth or gum issues, lying, tonsilitis, TMJ, lack of purpose, fear of speaking, Tourette syndrome	Vision problems, dyslexia, migraines, nightmares, bipolar, sleep disorders, sinus issues, hallucinations, lack of intuition	Alzheimer's, confusion, spaciness, mental illness, over-intellectualism, depression, apathy, Parkinson's, stroke, schizophrenia

MASCULINE AND FEMININE ENERGIES

To avoid any confusion on the topic of masculine and feminine energies, we first need to understand the different usages of these two terms. Yogis consider pure consciousness to be masculine, and call it "Shiva." Conversely, they consider the embodiment of Shiva consciousness and everything in the known physical world to be feminine, and call it "Shakti."

SHIVA AND SHAKTI

Shiva and Shakti are an indivisible pair representing universal energy, and everything that manifests out of that energy. In the highest meaning of the terms masculine and feminine, Shiva is the masculine, all-knowing god-energy that has no form, and Shakti is the feminine embodied form of Shiva. This means everything manifest, including our beautiful Mother Earth, is feminine in a general, Shakti sense.

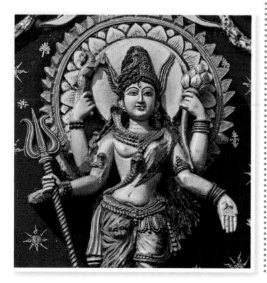

Still, within this physical world, it's very helpful to break everything down further into feminine and masculine polarities. This is particularly true when working with the chakras, because they alternate between yin and yang energy as they move up the spine.

"Yang" simply refers to masculine energy, which is contractive, strong, and self-contained. This kind of energy seeks to express itself through external goals and outward success. "Yin" is feminine energy; it is expansive, soft, and other-oriented. Yin seeks to express itself through rich inner experiences and meaningful relationships. Men and women carry equal amounts of these two types of energy in their spiritual essence. But gender, hormones, socialization, and personal beliefs start to create inequities in how these energies are experienced and expressed in our bodies. For this reason, masculine qualities seem to fit

This half Shiva–half Shakti deity from a temple in Puri, India, shows our innate masculine and feminine energies.

men more readily, and feminine qualities seem to be more easily found in women.

This distinction between masculine and feminine energies may seem complicated, but it's actually quite simple. Most of us have a really good, innate sense of which qualities are yin and which ones are yang.

Use the simple exercise below to test your intuitive sense of masculine and feminine energies.

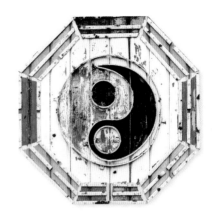

The feng shui bagua symbol with its yin–yang center represents perfect masculine–feminine balance.

IDENTIFYING MASCULINE AND FEMININE QUALITIES

Write the qualities listed below on a sheet of paper and put an M next to the words you feel are masculine and an F next to the ones you feel are feminine.

1. Strong	7. Motivated
2. Sensitive	8. Easy-going
3. Focused	9. Stable
4. Caring	10. Emotional
5. Purposeful	11. Powerful
6. Intuitive	12. Generous

If you put an M next to all of the odd-numbered qualities and an F next to all of the even-numbered characteristics, your understanding of masculine and feminine energies is exactly right.

THE PULSATION OF THE BODILY CHAKRAS

In that last exercise, the first six qualities are associated with each of the six embodied chakras like this:

1. **Strong** = Root
2. **Sensitive** = Sacral
3. **Focused** = Solar Plexus
4. **Caring** = Heart
5. **Purposeful** = Throat
6. **Intuitive** = Brow

The odd-numbered qualities are masculine and the even-numbered qualities are feminine. Because your chakras pulsate consistently between masculine and feminine energies, we're all innately set up for energetic, yin–yang balance. Still, navigating these polarities in a physical body can be challenging. One thing that really helps is being aware of the places in your body where these opposing energies meet.

THE CHAKRA NEXUS POINTS

Because the chakras alternate between masculine and feminine energy, the points between them provide an opportunity to practice balance. These powerful places where adjacent chakras meet are called the chakra nexus points.

The primary chakra nexus points are located:

- Between your root and sacral chakra (deep in your pelvis)
- Between your solar plexus and heart chakra (at the bottom of your heart)
- Between your throat and brow chakra (in the upper palate of your mouth)

The location of the two secondary chakra nexus points is:

- Between your sacral and solar plexus chakra (in your lower belly)
- Between your heart and throat chakra (in your high heart)

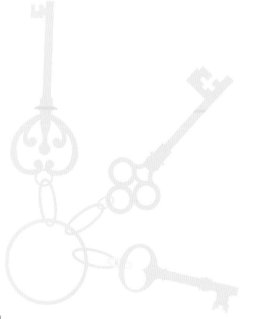

ROOT–SACRAL CHAKRA NEXUS POINT

These two are absolute opposites. The root chakra is masculine and related to stability and longevity (just like actual roots), while your sacral chakra is feminine and constantly changing like its element, water. Here are some key contrasting qualities you want to balance at the root–sacral nexus point:

ROOT	SACRAL
(Masculine)	*(Feminine)*
Strong	Flexible
Committed	Noncommittal
Planned	Spontaneous
Organized	Chaotic
Unmoving	Fluid

SOLAR PLEXUS–HEART CHAKRA NEXUS POINT

The solar plexus is a masculine chakra with self-oriented, warrior energy, and the heart is a feminine chakra of loving, expansive energy.

Our culture tends to embrace love, and reject anything "selfish," but the truth is, both of these energies are necessary. On the most basic level, if we don't love and care for ourselves, we're not healthy or strong enough to love and care for others. Here's what you need to balance at the solar plexus–heart nexus point:

SOLAR PLEXUS (Masculine)	HEART (Feminine)
Power	Love
Focus on self	Focus on others
Preferential love	Unconditional love
Creating transformation	Accepting what is
Confident	Humble

THROAT–BROW CHAKRA NEXUS POINT

The polarity between the energy of the throat and brow chakras is far less pronounced than the other two main chakra nexus points, because, as we get closer to the crown, fewer differences exist. In fact, in some ways, these two chakras are more similar than different. Still, there's enough of a masculine–feminine pulsation here to create these subtle contrasts:

THROAT (Masculine)	BROW (Feminine)
Personal perspective	Unbiased perspective
Outward expression	Inward introspection
Personal truth	Universal truth

The three primary chakra nexus points are important focal points in Hatha yoga. The secondary points are less essential.

SACRAL–SOLAR PLEXUS CHAKRA NEXUS POINT

The sacral chakra carries divine feminine energy that's flowing and easy going, whereas the solar plexus chakra holds the masculine energy of fire and action. Together, their elements—fire and water—can create steam, if you can balance these aspects:

SACRAL (Feminine)	SOLAR PLEXUS (Masculine)
Passive	Aggressive
Follow	Lead
Feeling	Thinking
Surrender	Fight
Allow	Make happen

HEART–THROAT CHAKRA NEXUS POINT

Again, we're getting closer to the crown, so these two energy centers are not as differentiated as the others. Still, here are a few qualities you can work on balancing:

HEART (Feminine)	THROAT (Masculine)
Kind and compassionate	"Brutally" honest
Gentle caretaker	Driven motivator
Loving what is	Creating growth

THE ENERGY CURRENTS OF YOUR BODY

Now that you understand the nature of your chakras and the chakra nexus points, we are ready to explore the bigger picture of how energy flows through your body. You're going to be amazed by the extent of your body's energy systems!

Your body has a complex network of energy channels that yogis call *nadis*. There are differing estimates of how many nadis exist in the body, but the favored number by yogis is 72,000. The term "nadi" is Sanskrit for "vein, river, or nerve," all of which are good metaphors for the invisible currents that move prana (energy) throughout your body.

Your chakras reside along your spinal column, at the places where most nadis intersect. To put it another way, if your body were a map, your nadis would be the roads, and your chakras would be the big cities into which most of the roads lead. Out of the thousands of nadis in your body, there really are only three key ones that yogis emphasize—the sushumna, the ida, and the pingala.

THE SUSHUMNA

The sushumna is that most important nadi of all. Just as the biggest cities tend to reside along one major railroad or highway, your chakras are lined up on the biggest and busiest energy current of your body, your sushumna, the vertical energy axis along your spine.

The word "sushumna" is Sanskrit for "a particular vein or artery" and also "gracious or kind." Indeed, this benevolent energy highway is quite good to all of us. It's the passageway that allows us to experience the full range of our existence from pure, spiritual energy at the crown, to total physical embodiment at the root. It's the ladder that we move up and down as we navigate being a spirit in a body.

THE IDA AND PINGALA

The ida and pingala are the feminine and masculine (moon and sun) energies that make their way up and down the sushumna through the chakras.

The ida is the cool, lunar energy that corresponds to feminine qualities like nurturing and introspection, and the pingala is the warm, solar energy that corresponds to masculine qualities like physical vitality and worldly pursuits.

The ida and pingala nadis begin at the root chakra and terminate at the bottom of the third-eye chakra. Some traditions believe that you cannot pierce the veil of the crown chakra if the ida and pingala are not balanced.

The breathing practice of Nadi Shodhana (also known as alternative nostril breathing) is widely considered the best way to balance your ida and pingala energies (see page 45).

If you look at an image of the ida and pingala nadis winding around the chakras, you may notice they look a lot like two well-known symbols: the caduceus of the medical world and the double helix pattern of our DNA. Even though allopathic or mainstream medicine has strayed far from the world of energy healing, the fact that its symbol, the caduceus, looks like a perfect replica of our energy field, seems to be at least a subconscious acknowledgment of the healing power of our chakras.

It's possible, also, that our DNA is a microcosmic slice of our energy field. Scientists used to believe that DNA was immutable, but are learning now that it changes. Since our energy field is constantly shifting, perhaps our DNA is a tiny snapshot of our energy blueprint at any given moment. The outer

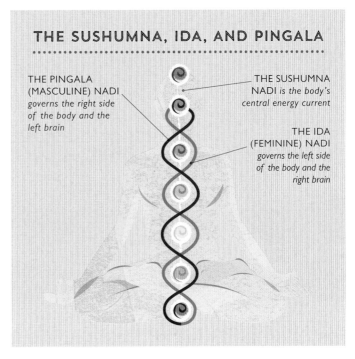

THE SUSHUMNA, IDA, AND PINGALA

THE PINGALA (MASCULINE) NADI *governs the right side of the body and the left brain*

THE SUSHUMNA NADI *is the body's central energy current*

THE IDA (FEMININE) NADI *governs the left side of the body and the right brain*

boundaries of our DNA look an awful lot like our ida and pingala energy channels.

Putting aside all theories for now, let's look at what we know about the way our energy moves in 3D, physical space.

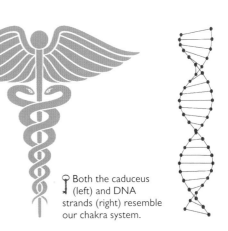

Both the caduceus (left) and DNA strands (right) resemble our chakra system.

THE ENERGY CURRENTS OF THREE-DIMENSIONAL SPACE

Y ou are spiritual energy moving in 3D space. In each of the three dimensions, there are two opposing forces. This means you are always working with the polarized aspects of these three important "dimensions" of energy for a total of six directions: Up–Down, Left–Right, and Front–Back.

THE ENERGY DIRECTIONS

Up–Down: Of the directional polarities, up–down is the most essential since it connects us to the realm of consciousness, and therefore to the Divine. The upward energy is called the Liberating Current, because it lightens us up; the downward channel is called the Manifesting Current, because it allows us to turn spiritual inspiration and ideas into manifest things. We'll talk more of these key currents in chapter two when we discuss the three main chakra types.

Left–Right: The left–right energy gives you the ability to be passive in a feminine way or active in a masculine way, with the left side of the body connecting to the feminine right hemisphere of the brain and the right side of the body connecting to the masculine left hemisphere of the brain.

Front–Back: The front–back energy gives us the ability to move forward or back in space, representing our future and past, as well as our conscious (front) and subconscious (back).

VORTEX ENERGY

If you look at the caduceus, you can see that the ida and pingala are winding around the central axis as if they're being pulled by all six of these dimensional forces at once—left and right, forward and back, up and down. From these natural forces, dynamic, vortex energy is created. It moves through all of the major endocrine gland areas and continually recreates and interacts with our chakras.

So the masculine–feminine balancing we've been discussing so far actually exists on these three different, directional planes. In chapter two, when we assess our chakras we will look at whether we are honoring the energy of our front and back, left and right, and, especially, our essential liberating and manifesting currents. We will also look at how our Western culture strongly favors masculine energy and how that bias affects our energy field.

BALANCING MASCULINE AND FEMININE ENERGIES

Nadi Shodhana (alternative nostril breathing) is the preferred practice for balancing the masculine (pingala) and feminine (ida) energies that move through your chakras. Practicing it for just a few moments a day will help balance your brain hemispheres and give you a better sense of energetic equilibrium.

1. Find a comfortable seated position.

2. Close your eyes and breathe normally for a few cycles.

3. When your breath feels natural, full, and relaxed, make the Vishnu mudra in your right hand. With your hand open, curl the tips of your index and middle finger inward until they touch the palm of your hand, like this:

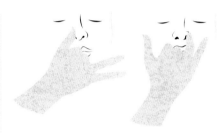

VISHNU MUDRA

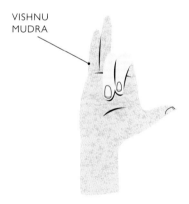

4. Keeping this hand position, press your right thumb down on your right nostril to close it, and exhale through your left nostril, as shown in the next illustration.

5. Now inhale through your left nostril, and at the top of the inhale, use your left ring finger to press down on your left nostril while you lift your thumb and exhale out your right nostril, as shown in the second illustration above.

6. Inhale fully through your right nostril and use your thumb to close the right nostril, as you lift your left ring finger and exhale out the left nostril.

7. Continue to alternate nostril breathing like this for several rounds, until you feel calmer and more balanced. Be sure to end by exhaling out the right nostril for balance.

NOTE: Some people prefer a slightly different hand position. Rather than curl their index and middle fingers, they extend them and rest them on the third-eye area.

ALL ABOUT YOUR AURA

Each of us has a biomagnetic field around us that is an energetic outgrowth of our chakras. This field is called an aura, and it contains our individual energy blueprint. Your aura is like an energetic calling card, because it's the first thing people sense when they meet you. It's the reason we have sayings like "he has an aura about him" or "she's glowing." Just like your fingerprint, your aura is unique to you. But unlike your fingerprint, your aura is continually shifting according to your emotions, health, and state of mind.

THE SEVEN LAYERS OF YOUR AURA

Your aura is comprised of seven layers, called subtle bodies, that are directly connected to each of your chakras.

The first three that are closest to the body—the etheric, emotional, and mental subtle bodies—represent your lower chakras and the physical realm.

The middle auric layer is connected to your heart chakra and serves as the gateway to the upper chakras and divine energies.

Your three outermost auric layers—the etheric template, celestial, and ketheric subtle bodies—represent your upper chakras and are related to the spiritual realm.

In other words, each layer vibrates at a higher rate as you move outward from the body, with the first layer connected to the root chakra having the slowest vibration, and the seventh layer connected to the crown vibrating the fastest.

THE SEVEN LAYERS OF THE AURA

CAUSAL BODY

CELESTIAL BODY

ETHERIC TEMPLATE

MENTAL BODY

ASTRAL BODY

EMOTIONAL BODY

ETHERIC BODY

AURIC LAYER #1 Etheric Body *(Root Chakra)*	The etheric body is the closest to your physical body and typically extends outward 1–3 inches (2.5–7.6cm). It is related to your root chakra and is primarily about your health and tribe, as well as your beliefs about both.
AURIC LAYER #2 Emotional Body *(Sacral Chakra)*	The emotional body resides about 2–3 inches (5–7.6cm) off the body and is related to your sacral chakra and all your emotions, including unprocessed feelings from the past. This layer shifts as your moods shift.
AURIC LAYER #3 Mental Body *(Solar Plexus Chakra)*	The mental body resides about 3–8 inches (7.6–20cm) off the body and is related to your solar plexus chakra and all your mental processes, ideas, and judgments. This layer is connected to both the conscious and subconscious mind, and will reveal any self-doubts or limiting beliefs.
AURIC LAYER #4 Astral Body *(Heart Chakra)*	The astral body typically spreads out to about 1 foot off the body and is related to the heart chakra. It represents our feelings of peace, love, and connection to others and will reveal if we have grief or a hardened heart.
AURIC LAYER #5 Etheric Template *(Throat Chakra)*	The etheric template usually extends from about 1½–2 feet (0.5–0.6m) from the body and is related to the throat chakra. It is where all manifestation begins. The "template" in the name of this body refers to the spiritual blueprint that outlines everything that will manifest into the world through the etheric plane.
AURIC LAYER #6 Celestial Body *(Brow Chakra)*	The celestial aura layer is normally about 2–2½ feet (0.6–0.8m) off the body and is related to the third-eye chakra. It's associated with higher perception and intuition, and an unconditional love for all beings everywhere.
AURIC LAYER #7 Causal Body *(Crown Chakra)*	The causal layer typically extends out as far as 3 feet (0.9m) and is related to the crown chakra. This layer vibrates more quickly than all the others. It holds all the information about all lifetimes, and imparts a deep knowing and sense of unity with everything.

SENSING AND SEEING AURAS

Some people who are sensitive or clairvoyant can actually see auras. But seeing them isn't the only way to experience them. Most people intuitively feel others' auras. This is good because our aura is the most accurate representation of who we truly are at any given moment in time. It relays information about our mind, emotions, physical health, and even any past traumas that haven't been fully resolved.

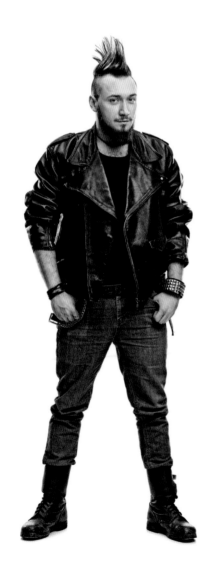

FIRST IMPRESSIONS

Anyone can manipulate the way they appear, but no one can fake their auric energy. For instance, a person can wear bold clothes to seem more confident, or put on a smile to seem happier, but there is no way to shift your aura to make it something it's not. It always reveals the truth, and this makes it the most accurate measure of your true state of being. This is why first impressions can be so powerful, and why they often have nothing to do with appearances.

We've all experienced occasions when we have immediately distrusted someone who appeared trustworthy, or conversely, trusted a stranger who looked quite suspect. Certainly outward appearances were not what we were using to base our judgment. Instead, we were "reading" the other person's auric field, feeling how theirs "fit" with ours, and using our intuition to size them up.

Our intuitive sense of another's aura is part of what gives us a particular first impression.

SENSING AURAS

Here's a simple way to feel another's aura and also learn about the size of your own.

1. Ask a few friends (four or more) to do an auric exercise with you. Go outside and find a large, open, and preferably quiet space.

2. Have your first friend stand 100 feet (30 m) away from you and turn your back.

3. Close your eyes and allow yourself to become open and sensitive to any and all energetic sensations.

4. Ask your friend to walk toward you very slowly. When you feel him or her in your field, say "Stop!"

5. Turn round and see how far your friend is from you, measure the space between the two of you and write it down. This is the spot where your two auras meet.

6. Do the same with your other friends, and then figure out the average of all the stop points you measured. Divide it by two (since both your auras are meeting), and this should give you a really good idea of the size of your aura.

7. Allow each of your friends to take your place as the primary and feel into their stop points too, so they can determine their aura sizes as well.

EXTENDED AURAS

A healthy aura typically extends about 18 inches (45.7 cm) to 3 feet (0.9 m) from the body, but people who have had a lot of trauma in their life may have a much bigger aura, even as far as 50 feet (15 m) off their body. This is due to the fact that they have felt unsafe in the world and have habitually sent their energy outward like a sentinel to see if a situation is dangerous.

An easy way to detect if someone has an overly expanded aura is to ask them how they feel in a crowd. People with a really big aura will typically feel overwhelmed in the midst of a lot of people, because they are sensing the energies of all the different people who are inside their large auric field at the same time.

WHAT DOES AN AURA LOOK LIKE?

Most diagrams of auras show a cross-section view (like the one on page 46), as if the aura has been cut in half. In this way, you can see the various "layers" that relate to each chakra.

But for those who can see auras, they don't look this way. Rather than seeing a cross section, they see all the layers of the auras shining through at once.

Aura photos use biofeedback to give you a representation of what your aura looks like.

Typically, because some layers are stronger than others, different colors may dominate different areas. If one auric layer is stronger than the others, that color will shine through more than the rest, and the whole aura may come off as a shade of that color.

It's important to keep in mind that each layer includes all the others inside of it that are closer to the body. This means the seventh ketheric layer includes all the others, and any aura diagrams containing discrete layers are good for educational purposes, but are not really representative of the way the aura actually looks.

KEYNOTE

In general, young children are more able than adults to see auras, because they have not yet learned to restrict their vision to the "normal" range. You may notice that babies often look above your head, or just beyond your body's outline when gazing at you. This is their way of taking all of you in, especially your auric field, because it's so stimulating and colorful.

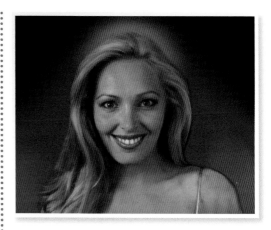

AURA PHOTOS

If you want to get a photo of your aura, you should be aware that, currently, there is no apparatus that can actually take a picture of it. The photos you buy in a new-age store or at a fair are actually reproductions of what a biofeedback system thinks your aura looks like. Typically, the reading comes from temperature or acupressure measurements taken from the fingers of one hand. The two times I've had aura photos taken, they've seemed pretty accurate.

So how do they work? Well, there are yogic and Ayurvedic traditions that connect particular fingers to each chakra element (earth, water, fire, etc.). And heat and pressure can be reliable indicators of human energy, so it's quite possible that measuring these things could create a decent representation of your aura. In any case, aura photos are fun, and they make a great souvenir!

EYE TRAINING FOR SEEING AURAS

If you want to see your own or another's aura, your best bet is to retrain your eyes to see them. First, you need to sensitize your eye muscles to a wider, visual spectrum. Here's a good exercise for doing that:

1. Get a few sheets of construction paper in red, green, blue, and yellow. Cut out some basic geometric shapes—e.g. a triangle, square, rectangle, and circle—each one about 3–4 inches (7.6–10 cm) square.

2. Paste each shape onto separate sheets of white paper.

3. Stare at one of these geometric shapes for about 30 seconds, then remove the paper and look at a blank sheet of paper. You will see a "shadow image" of the original shape. It will be the same shape and size, but the opposite, complementary color.

4. Keep looking at this shadow image until it disappears. Notice how soft the image is as it fades away. This is what it is like to see an aura. You are totally focused, but remain soft in your perception.

Doing this exercise will ready your eyes for seeing actual auras, if your mind is open to seeing them. When you have done this exercise for at least a week, you can start trying to see actual auras by taking the following steps:

1. Have a friend stand before a white wall.

2. Step back about 8 feet (2.5m) and focus on the middle of his or her body (around the solar plexus).

3. Keep your eyes fixed on this focal spot, but relax them and begin to notice the body's outline with your peripheral vision.

Any perception of an outline around the body is an indicator that you are starting to see the aura. You may see only a light outline at first, no color. Try not to judge or push things at this point. Just continue to practice working with this relaxed vision. Eventually, you will begin to see colors. You're building new muscles and brain pathways here, so be patient and curious, and it will come.

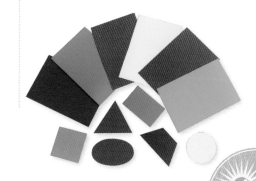

AURA COLOR MEANINGS

There are many different interpretations of what the different aura colors mean, because words are far more limited than colors, and there is an endless variety of possible hues that we label as one color. Nevertheless, it's fun to endeavor to find meaning in the infinite spectrum of possible colors within us. Here is a list of some of the more commonly accepted meanings for the most basic aura colors:

- **Red:** Committed, career-oriented, independent, protector
- **Red-Orange:** Sexual, vibrant, maverick, manifestor
- **Orange:** Creative, productive, adventurous, entertainer
- **Orange-Yellow:** Emotionally intelligent, secure, systematic, problem-solver
- **Yellow:** Intelligent, optimistic, confident, leader
- **Yellow-Green:** Happy, balanced, generous, humanitarian
- **Green:** Unconditionally loving, gentle, open-minded, caregiver
- **Pink:** Sensitive, unique, romantic, innovator

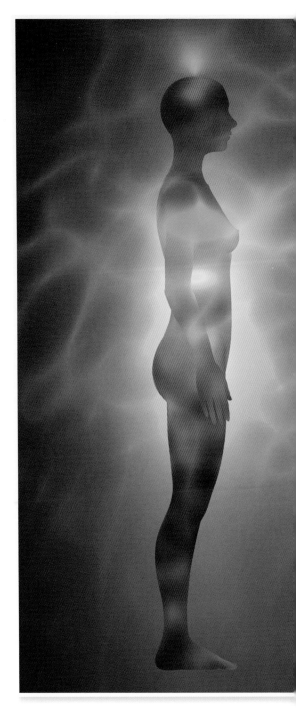

This image shows all the chakra colors but, typically, your aura will be a single color or duo blend.

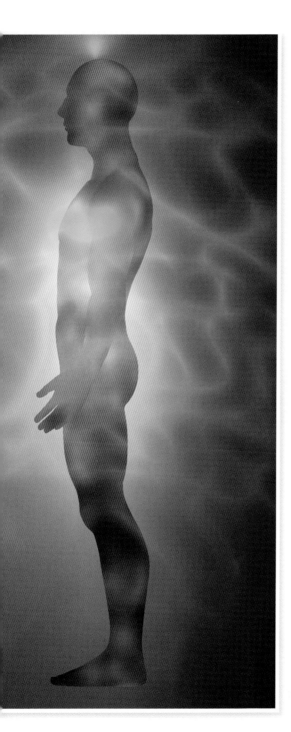

- **Turquoise:** Communicative, insightful, sharing, healer
- **Blue:** Gregarious, helpful, honest, teacher
- **Indigo:** Intuitive, wise, psychic, visionary
- **Violet:** Magical, spiritual, futuristic, idealist
- **Silver:** Spiritually connected, abundant, energetically strong
- **Gold:** Gifted, wise, light, guarded by spiritual beings
- **White:** Divine, peaceful, pure, transcendent being

In general, the presence of black indicates holding onto negative feelings due to unwillingness to forgive, and it's usually a sign of disease in the body. Other dark colors like gray or murky brown can indicate blockages, fears, and limitations.

THE ENDOCRINE SYSTEM AND THE CHAKRAS

Because most people cannot see the chakras, they sometimes doubt that they actually influence us physically, until they see how seamlessly they tie into the endocrine system. This system is the collection of glands that produce hormones, which in turn regulate many important bodily functions, including mood, sleep, metabolism, and growth.

The chakras may be energetic, but they consistently create very real, physical changes in our bodies, because each chakra stimulates at least one of our ductless glands that is located right near it. That gland then sends out chemical messengers that keep our body functioning properly and in harmony with our nervous system.

This explains why a "map" of our endocrine system looks quite similar to our chakra system, with each ductless gland lining up with one chakra, as shown in the box below. As the illustration of the two systems shows, the relationship is direct and symmetrical.

THE ENDOCRINE GLANDS AND THE CHAKRAS

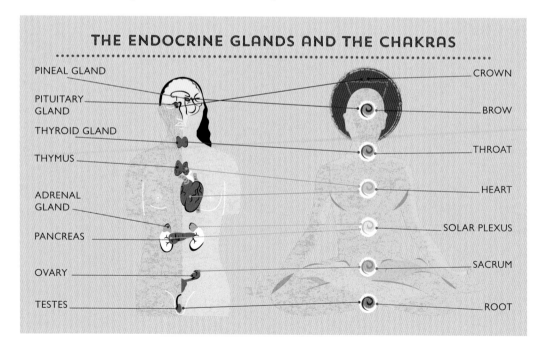

PINEAL GLAND — CROWN

PITUITARY GLAND — BROW

THYROID GLAND

THYMUS — THROAT

ADRENAL GLAND — HEART

PANCREAS — SOLAR PLEXUS

OVARY — SACRUM

TESTES — ROOT

A NOTE ABOUT ROOT AND SACRAL CHAKRA ASSOCIATIONS

As the illustration shows, the relationship between the chakras and their related glands is direct. Each endocrine gland is in the area of the chakra that affects it.

For some reason, over the years, the root chakra has become wrongly associated with the adrenals, which are actually in the solar plexus area, and the sacral chakra has been mistakenly associated with the testes, which are located in the root chakra's domain.

If we accept the fact that the vortex energy of each chakra stimulates the endocrine glands that are closest to it, we also have to embrace the idea that women do not have the glands that are affected by root chakra energy (the testes), and that men do not have the glands that are influenced by the energy of the second chakra (the ovaries).

This interpretation actually works, but in order to explain it, we need to talk about the sexual nature of our chakras, and the different ways that men and women experience their sexuality.

CHAKRAS AND SEXUALITY

There has been a good deal of disagreement among chakra scholars about the energetic location of human sexuality. Some say it's in the root, and others say it's in the sacral chakra.

The confusion is most likely due to the fact that our sexuality is actually in both our first and second chakras and their related glands—the testes and ovaries. The experience of sex encompasses very different aspects, depending on your gender. If you have any doubt of this, just ask any man or woman about their sex life. You'll get two very different perspectives!

When it comes to sex, there's a masculine aspect that reflects first chakra energy and relates to procreation, physical release, and the survival of one's lineage. And there's an almost opposite, feminine aspect related to the sacral chakra that emphasizes intimacy, emotional connection, and pleasure.

In an ideal scenario, each gender can experience and enjoy both types of sex. Still, most men biologically carry more of the masculine energy and most women more of the feminine, due to the fact that the testes are stimulated by root chakra energy and the ovaries are influenced by sacral chakra energy.

THE ROOT CHAKRA

GLAND: TESTES

The testes produce testosterone, which gives men more libido, muscle strength, and bone density—all related to the root chakra.

Testosterone also makes male sexuality very physically oriented. For younger men especially, having sex and releasing semen is a very real, physical need. Of course, most men enjoy being intimate with, and emotionally connected to, their sexual partner too. Still, it's usually a secondary, rather than a primary, motivation, that awakens more as men age and their fertility declines.

The root chakra is often wrongly associated with the adrenal glands, which are little glands on top of each kidney that create the hormone adrenaline that springs us into action when we feel threatened. Associating the slowest, most stable chakra with the gland that gives us our "get up and go" is a mistake.

The root chakra carries the downward (apana) energy that allows us to relax—even sleep. It can't trigger us into quick action. That's the job of the third chakra.

THE SACRAL CHAKRA

GLAND: OVARIES

The sacral chakra is about sexuality, sensuality, fertility, intimacy, pleasure, and emotions. Unsurprisingly, the primary endocrine glands associated with this chakra are the female gonads, the ovaries.

The ovaries release the hormones and eggs that cause menstruation, and allow a woman to become pregnant and bear children. Those hormones also create a 28-day, feminine "moon cycle" that causes a woman's emotions to shift and fluctuate.

While men can obviously feel emotions and desire intimacy, they don't have the hormones that biologically predispose them to the menstrually-related emotional fluctuations women experience.

Because the testes put out root chakra hormones (testosterone) and the ovaries put out sacral chakra hormones (estrogen and progesterone), there is a natural sexual polarity between men and women. The second chakra is the realm of this kind of magnetic polarity, because it is all about partnering and creating intimacy.

THE SOLAR PLEXUS CHAKRA

GLAND: ADRENALS (PANCREAS)

The primary glands that are associated with the solar plexus are the adrenals. They reside on the top of our kidneys, right in the middle of the area governed by our third chakra. They put out adrenaline that triggers our "fight or flight" response, an automatic, physiological reaction of wanting to do battle or flee that occurs when we experience a perceived harmful event, attack, or threat.

In other words, the adrenals make us want to take action, which is the primary quality of the solar plexus. And they are even yellow!

Because the third chakra is also about digestion, and processing food for energy, it has a secondary endocrine gland, the pancreas. It secretes a variety of substances essential to effective digestion and also creates insulin, which helps to regulate the body's blood sugar level.

THE HEART CHAKRA

GLAND: THYMUS (HEART)

The thymus gland, which is located behind the sternum and between the lungs, creates white T-cells and specializes in immunity. Unlike most glands, it reaches its largest size in puberty and then begins to shrink, turning into a small globule of fat by late adulthood. By then, it has already created most of the T-cells we need for life.

Even though we have historically relegated the heart to the status of a mere blood-pumping organ, science has shown us that it is also an endocrine gland. In the mid-1980s, researchers found that the heart secretes hormones like the other endocrine glands. Perhaps we are so used to seeing the heart as an organ and universal symbol of love that we can't fully honor its role as an endocrine gland. It releases three different types of hormones that regulate blood pressure and promote cardiovascular health.

The other heart chakra gland, the thymus, gives us the immunity we need to be able to safely connect with others—one of the primary purposes of the heart chakra.

THE THROAT CHAKRA

 GLAND: THYROID
The thyroid gland is situated in front of the windpipe, just below the larynx. It takes iodine from food and creates two hormones that regulate the way the body uses energy. When this regulation works well, our metabolism is good. When it fails, we can experience hypothyroidism, where we are getting too little thyroid hormones, resulting in our feeling tired, sluggish, or, sometimes with children, growth is inhibited. Or, the other possible imbalance is hyperthyroidism, where the body overproduces thyroid hormones, resulting in a too-quick metabolism that causes anxiety, rapid heartbeat, hand tremors, etc.

It is interesting that the thyroid hormones are all about energy and growth because the purpose of the fifth chakra is "to grow" in the highest sense of the word. It is also quite fitting that the throat chakra regulates our energy levels, because it is the highest of the three masculine chakras (1, 3, and 5), which are all related to our ability to take action in the world.

THE BROW CHAKRA

 GLAND: PINEAL
Because the pineal gland is situated slightly higher in the brain than the pituitary, it is often falsely associated with the crown chakra, when in fact it is stimulated by the brow chakra (aka the third eye).

The pineal gland makes melatonin when it perceives light, the "element" that is related to the brow chakra. And it literally demonstrates a "sixth sense" by sensing light that shines not just on the eye area, but anywhere on the body. It seems the pineal can "see without eyes."

Even more fascinating is the fact that some lower vertebrates actually have a well-developed eye-like structure where their pineal gland is, which some scientists consider to be the evolutionary forerunner of the modern eye.

THE CROWN CHAKRA

GLAND: PITUITARY (HYPOTHALAMUS)

 The crown chakra and the pituitary are a perfect fit. Just as the seventh chakra is the master chakra, the pituitary is the master gland that regulates all the other glands. It does so with the aid of the hypothalamus. Together, these two glands produce the following key hormones:

- **Adrenocorticotropic hormone (ACTH)** that stimulates the adrenal glands to produce hormones, and **Growth hormone (GH)** that aids in creating healthy bones, muscle mass, and proper fat distribution (root chakra)
- **Follicle-stimulating hormone (FSH)** and **Luteinizing hormone (LH)** that work to ensure normal functioning of the ovaries and testes (sacral chakra)
- **ACTH** that stimulates the adrenal glands (solar plexus chakra)
- **Prolactin** that stimulates breast-milk production (heart chakra)
- **Thyroid-stimulating hormone** that prompts the thyroid gland to produce hormones (throat chakra)

Now that you have a more complete understanding of the chakras on both an energetic and a physical level, you are ready to assess the current state of your own chakras.

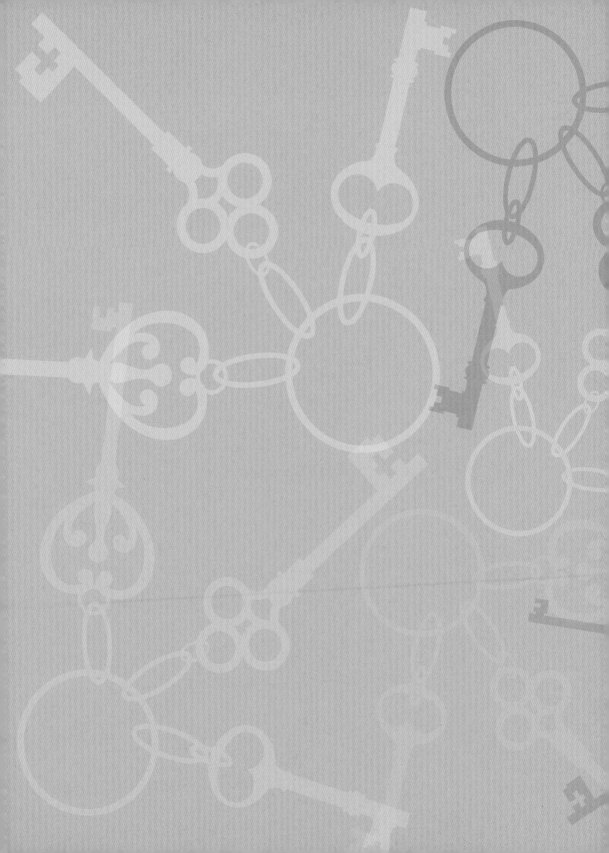

CHAPTER TWO

THE KEY
to
ASSESSING
YOUR
CHAKRAS

⚷ Uncover Your Essential Chakra
Needs and How to Get Them Fulfilled

⚷ Take Simple Written Tests to
Determine the Strength of Your Chakras

⚷ Find Out which Illnesses and
Diseases Relate to Each Chakra

THE IMPORTANCE OF ASSESSING YOUR CHAKRAS

One of the most common mistakes people make when working with their chakras is jumping right into "healing" without doing any diagnostics. A man might decide, for instance, that he wants to increase his psychic abilities, so he starts doing healing techniques that are purported to expand his third eye. Or he might feel he wants more money, so he starts working on his root chakra.

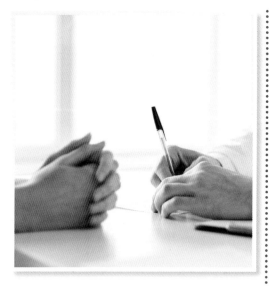

It's essential to get an assessment of your chakras before beginning any healing process.

And your doctor would never give you a treatment protocol or a prescription without first asking you some questions, giving you a physical exam, and doing any necessary blood work or tests.

Similarly, most exercise programs tell you to consult a doctor before you start, because even something generally positive like exercise can, in the wrong circumstance, be "bad." If you have a weak heart and jump right into a high cardio workout you risk giving yourself a heart attack. Or, if you're anorexic and you begin a high-calorie burning program, you could be harming yourself more than helping.

While there is nothing wrong with desiring to improve certain areas of your life through chakra healing, diving into healing before you understand the current state of your chakras is a misguided approach because shifting one chakra affects them all.

You wouldn't dream of walking into your doctor's office and telling her what treatment or prescription you wanted without first getting a diagnosis.

Even the most innocuous attempts at healing before getting an accurate assessment can do more harm than good, regardless of whether we're talking about physical or energetic healing.

ASSESSING YOURSELF IN A LOVING, SUPPORTIVE WAY

It's not only imperative that you assess your chakras, but that you do so in a loving, nonjudgmental way that keeps your heart and mind open.

When you assess your chakras, it's quite normal to find that certain ones are underactive or overactive. So you need to remember that you are already spiritually whole and you always will be. You aren't trying to "fix" yourself or become someone different. Rather, you are simply trying to experience your innate state of spiritual wholeness in an embodied way.

Think of your chakras as seven beautiful rooms in your spiritual mansion. You own this mansion free and clear. Nobody can

Your chakras are like seven elegant rooms in your spiritual mansion, just waiting to be opened.

take it away from you. Your seven lovely rooms will always exist. But do you have access to each and every room? Or are some of them locked? Are others so full of old family heirlooms that you can't get the door open? Chakra balancing gives you the keys to every room of your mansion so you can inhabit all of yourself.

With chakra work, you're not doing self-improvement, because you aren't trying to change yourself. Rather, you are simply becoming more yourself by stripping away habits, patterns, and belief systems that *aren't* you.

Our culture has a "fix it" mentality, so it's easy to fall into the improvement paradigm that fosters self-judgment. There's no reason ever to feel bad about your chakra assessments. They simply provide a temporary snapshot of your energy field, which is always changing.

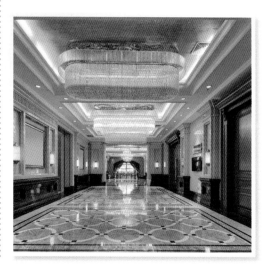

This snapshot, when looked at lovingly, can show you how to open your entire energetic field. It can also help you discover your biggest challenges, lessons, and gifts, if you can embrace them fully. So please be gentle and patient with yourself as you uncover your energetic patterns and blockages. Greet them with love and acceptance, and they will gradually shift. Judging yourself never leads to greater expansion, but nurturing yourself always supports you in becoming more of who you truly are.

THE GOAL IS TO BALANCE

You don't want to endeavor to heal an individual chakra until you have an understanding of its current relationship to all the other chakras, because your body's energy centers never operate in isolation. They are a system, and must be assessed and treated as a whole. This is not to say that you can't focus your healing on one particular chakra, because you absolutely can. Focusing on a single chakra is a great way of heightening the healing impact through concentrated action and intention.

But before you focus on a single chakra, you need to diagnose all seven to ensure that boosting one particular chakra will take you closer to, rather than farther away from, balancing your entire energy field.

PERSONAL AND PLANETARY ENERGIES ARE SHIFTING

Another common mistake people make when setting out to heal their chakras is thinking they need to focus on ascending their energy upward in order to reach "enlightenment." While this used to be true, the energies on our planet are rapidly shifting and changing the game. Thousands of years ago, when yogis first identified the chakras and began doing healing work, our planet was far more energetically heavy. The root chakra energy of stability ruled Earth. Marriages and careers lasted a lifetime, and caste systems lasted even longer than that.

Gravity was so predominant that the main goal of spiritual and energetic practices was to move upward in order to feel lighter and freer. Understandably, most yogis at the time focused on opening their upper chakras and getting their kundalini (stored root energy) to awaken and rise upward.

But we live in very different times now. Many people in the modern world lack grounding and are already quite open in their upper chakras. Some people even come into this planet with spiritual gifts already developed, and there are enough of them these days that we even have labels. We call them "indigo children," highly sensitive, or autistic. Some we even diagnose as ADHD!

You can tell that the root chakra energy is no longer such a dominant force on our planet, because there is far less stability than there was a century ago. Today, about half of all marriages end in divorce, most people pursue several different careers in their lifetime, and many of us move our domicile dozens of times.

Because of these planetary shifts, we can no longer assume that ascending up the chakras, or focusing on boosting the upper chakras, is the way to heal. For many people, there is a greater need to focus on grounding and moving energy downward. This is why practices like earthing (connecting to the earth for more vibrant health) are growing in popularity. The bottom line is this: The goal of chakra healing is to balance your energy field, and the best way to balance your chakras is to cultivate the energy of each chakra until they are all equally robust, open, and strong.

To do this, you must first measure the state of all your chakras and see which ones need boosting, and in rare cases, which ones need reducing. Once you've done this, you can engage in healing practices that are perfectly suited to balancing your entire energy field.

It's also important to keep in mind that you need to diagnose your chakras fairly often, because they are spinning vortices that are always in flux, and can shift in any moment. They may sometimes seem pretty immutable, because our belief systems and habit patterns keep them in the same underactive or overactive states. But in truth, they are continually changing, so try not to make any assumptions about where they are at any given time.

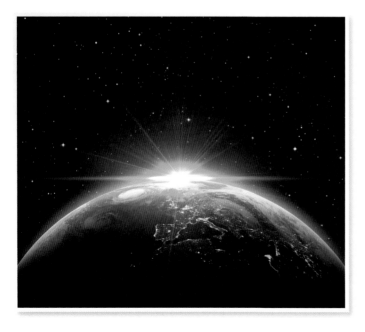

As the energies of our planet rise, some of us need to practice grounding and embodiment.

ASSESSING THE BALANCE OF YOUR THREE-DIMENSIONAL ENERGIES

One way to assess your chakras is to look at the way you balance the polarities of 3-D space. When you are perfectly balanced in all your chakras, vital energy flows up and down your shushumna, the energy current that moves through the center of your being. It also flows in the other two dimensions of space—forward and backward, as well as left and right.

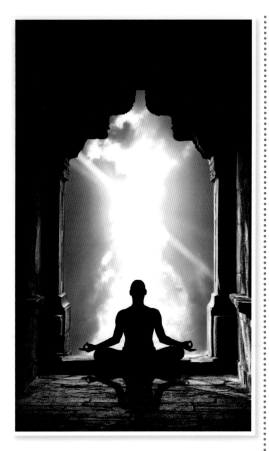

Yogis seek to balance their three-dimensional polarities to experience the chakra energy in their midline.

We looked at these oppositional pairs in chapter one. Here they are broken down into their energetic type:

Masculine	Feminine
Up ("Shiva")	Down ("Shakti")
Front	Back
Right	Left

If you can perfectly balance these polarities, you end up with energy moving dynamically up and down the midline of your body in the same way as when your chakras are fully balanced.

You can actually see this if you look at a diagram showing your body separated into front–back, right–left, up–down sections (see facing page).

The common point is the line that runs right through your chakras. For this reason, paying attention to these key pairs of polar energy is a good alternative way to bring more balance to your chakras.

WESTERN WORLD ENERGY BIAS

When assessing whether you are balancing these energetic pairs, it's important to realize that in the West, we tend to prefer and emphasize the masculine over the feminine.

In general, we think it's better to "ascend" or "be enlightened" than it is to be "down" or "descending." We think moving forward is better than going backward, and, in the English language, we call one of our hands "right" (meaning "correct") and the other "left" (as in "what's left"). In French the word for left is "gauche," which carries a negative connotation and means awkward, clumsy, or unhappy.

I mention this simply so you can be aware that most of us in the Western world are imbalanced toward our masculine side. And if we are outside the norm and actually more feminine, we may judge ourselves and thwart our power in an attempt not to seem too different.

Being aware of this cultural tendency helps you to seek out and heal the subconscious ways in which you may be avoiding your feminine energy or making it wrong.

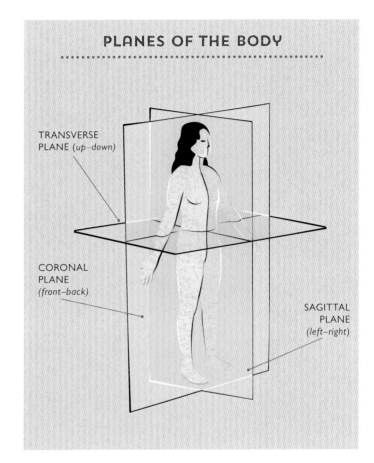

PLANES OF THE BODY

TRANSVERSE PLANE (*up–down*)

CORONAL PLANE (*front–back*)

SAGITTAL PLANE (*left–right*)

ARE YOUR CHAKRAS "OPEN" OR "CLOSED?"

Because your chakras are little energy vortices that act like revolving doors, people often refer to them as "open" or "closed." I sometimes do this too, in order to communicate in already familiar terms, and for the sake of verbal variety. But let's be very clear, your chakras are not a binary system of open or closed. They exist on a spectrum of openness, which means it's more accurate and useful to think of them as being barely open, kind of open, and very open. There really is no such thing as a totally "closed" chakra, at least not while we're still alive. Even if a chakra is very sluggish and barely open, it's still not 100 percent "closed."

Rather than using these inaccurate, binary terms, consider selecting words that allow for more range, for example, "underactive" or "overactive." The advantage of choosing these words is two-fold: first, they are prescriptive by nature, because if a chakra is underactive, you want to make it more active, and if it's overactive, you want to make it less active; and second they are relatively neutral and nonjudgmental descriptions. They allow us to diagnose without using negative, potentially restrictive labels that might limit our growth.

There are other terms like "excessive" and "deficient" or "weak," which are more accurate than open or closed, but have a downside of carrying a slightly negative connotation that might invite self-judgment and subconsciously sabotage the healing process.

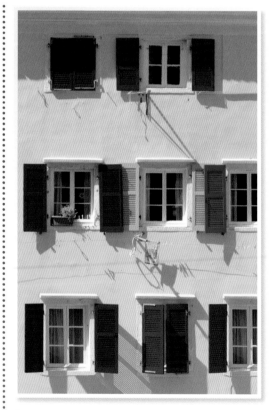

Just like shutters on windows, your chakras can have different degrees of openness.

For variety, I occasionally use all of these terms, but I find that in general, the words "open" and "closed" are the least accurate, whereas "underactive" and "overactive" are the most prescriptively useful.

UNDERACTIVE OR OVERACTIVE?

The key thing to remember when using the terms "underactive" and "overactive" is that they are relative, depending on the strength of your whole chakra system. For instance, if on a scale of 0–10 (where 0 means a chakra is totally closed and 10 means it is completely open), and six of your chakras were rated a 6, but your solar plexus chakra was rated a 9, then it would be relatively overactive, because it is dwarfing the others.

But if, on that same scale, all your chakras were rated a 9, then a solar plexus with a 9 rating would not be overactive, but normal. You would simply have a super-boosted, very balanced chakra system. Likewise, if all of your chakras were rated very low, you could have very balanced, underactive chakras. In this case, being "balanced" would not necessarily be a healthy state, since we need a certain amount of energy moving through our system.

In other words, in order to know if a chakra is underactive or overactive, you must know the openness of *all* your chakras.

Your chakras are relative like these lightbulbs. If one is much stronger than the others, it is overactive.

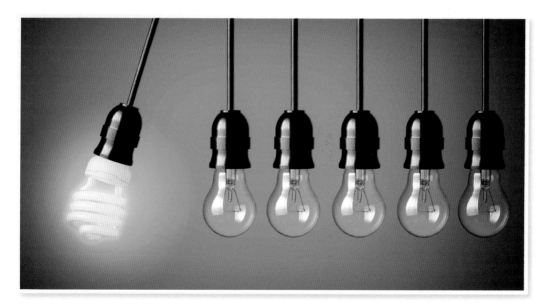

WHAT CREATES CHAKRA WEAKNESS?

As spiritual beings, we have a strong, energetic tendency toward wholeness. Why then, do we experience weakness in certain chakras? What causes us to get out of balance?

YOUR PAST LIFE EXPERIENCES

Energy never dies. It just changes form. This means, as spiritual beings, we never truly die. We simply reincarnate into a different body. Our human identity changes, but our soul maintains continuity across our many lifetimes.

For this reason, we are not an energetic "blank slate" when we're born. We bring in clear tendencies and predilections. This is why we see amazing child prodigies who come into this world with masterful skills they were never taught, and are too young to have learned.

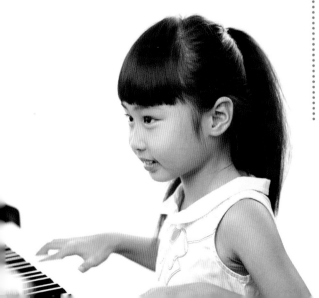

Similarly, our soul brings chakra imbalances into each lifetime. Many people believe we actually incarnate in order to heal these imbalances, limitations, or fears, so we can come to know our true, unlimited nature.

In any case, your soul's "memories" are one potential cause of chakra weakness.

YOUR ANCESTORS' EXPERIENCES

Just as your soul has memories from other lives, your body does too. Except in this case, the other lives were not yours, but those of your ancestors. Your genes actually hold a record of all the things your relatives have ever experienced. And since modern life is far more convenient than days of old, it's safe to assume that your genes are carrying a lot of the hardships and fears your ancestors experienced.

♀ When children show unfathomable prodigious talents, it's likely those skills came from a past life.

The scientific community has begun to show this. In one very fascinating study, researchers subjected mice to shock while exposing them to a particular scent, and eventually the mice became afraid when exposed to the scent without any shocks occurring. But that's not the interesting part. The researchers then exposed the offspring of the rodents to the same scent, and although the offspring had never been conditioned by shock, they displayed a marked fear response to the scent.

And in the realm of human studies, research on children who were conceived during a harsh wartime famine in the Netherlands in the 1940s revealed that they had an increased risk of diabetes, heart disease, and other serious health conditions, possibly because of epigenetic alterations to genes involved in these diseases. From these studies we can conclude that your genes are quite literally carrying energetic propensities that are related to your ancestors' experiences.

YOUR CURRENT LIFE EXPERIENCES

While you have undoubtedly brought energetic tendencies into the world, most likely the biggest influence on your chakra energy has been your own life experiences, particularly those of your early childhood.

From the age of one to seven, your foundational root chakra forms. During this time, you're learning how to live in a body and get your basic needs met. (See pages 72–77 for an exploration of your basic chakra needs.)

Each of your chakras has a basic need, and as each need is met in a healthy way, the foundation is built for the related chakra to be naturally strong and open.

YOUR WEAKNESSES ARE YOUR STRENGTHS

As you assess your chakras, please keep one thing in mind: your most profound gifts are the things you've learned from your own struggles.

When you're a healer, your problems are gifts, because they challenge you to heal yourself and find your own way. Only after you have made your way out of your own metaphorical jungle can you then be a guide for others.

In my case, almost all my problems were root chakra issues, so I had to find ways to ground and connect with the Earth. After years of doing it, I now teach others to do the same. I guarantee that your biggest chakra weaknesses will morph into your most revered strengths, if you continually commit to healing yourself and to doing the necessary work.

THE FIRST SEVEN YEARS: YOUR BASIC CHAKRA NEEDS

Here is a breakdown of the basic needs that must be met in each of the first seven years of life.

AGE 1—ROOT:
THE NEED FOR SAFETY

At a foundational level, we all need to feel safe and secure, and this need is particularly predominant from the time we are born through age one.

During this period, we are learning to live in a body, and to get our survival needs met. This means we are paying attention to and trying to abide by the rules and beliefs of our extended family, so we can create a safe, reliable atmosphere for ourselves.

For this reason, safety is the primary need of our root chakra and creating stability is a related, secondary need.

How safe and stable were the first couple years of your life? Did your family live in one place or move around? Were there any major changes like death, divorce, or some other sort of substantial loss?

How important are safety and stability to you now? Think about it. What have you done in the past to keep things in your comfort zone or to stick with what you're already familiar with? What would you do in the future to avoid radical change and keep the status quo?

This first chakra need often gets met by remaining in a situation, like a love relationship or a job, well past its natural expiration date.

On a positive note, our need for safety causes us to stick with things, so we can be loyal to the people and careers we love and become masterful at the activities that interest us.

AGE 2—SACRAL:
THE NEED FOR VARIETY

The need of the second chakra is the opposite of the first because, as we discovered in chapter one, the root and sacral chakras are polarized masculine–feminine energies.

Once we humans feel stable and safe, we get bored stiff if that's all there is! We also need things to be a bit unstable. In other words, we need things to change. This means the primary need of the sacral chakra is variety, the so-called "spice of life."

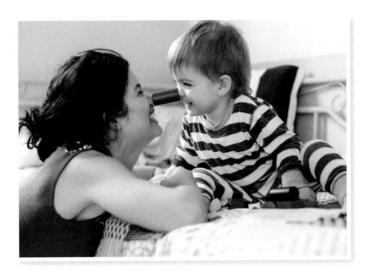

Two-year olds need playful, emotionally rich relationships with their caregivers.

home, relationship, or job, prematurely or too often. Within a relationship, this need might also be met through infidelity, particularly if someone is trying to meet both their first and second chakra needs simultaneously. Their need for stability keeps them in their committed relationship, while their need for variety compels them to have someone else on the side.

The positive aspect of our need for variety is that it keeps us young and flexible as we seek new ways of being and take on novel pursuits.

As a small child, one of the main ways this variety shows up is in the everyday playful, creative interactions we share with our caregivers. This is why intimacy is a key secondary need of the sacral chakra.

How was your relationship with your caregivers when you were two years old? Did they play with you and show you that it was okay to feel and express the full range of your emotions?

How important are variety and change to you? What have you done in the past to create variety in your life? To shake things up and move away from the "same old, same old?" What would you do in the future to avoid monotony and to create more spice in your life?

This second chakra need often gets met by leaving situations, for example a

AGE 3—SOLAR PLEXUS: THE NEED FOR SIGNIFICANCE

The need of the third chakra is significance which is related to our sense of personal power. During the period when we are approaching our third birthday, we begin to access the fiery energy of our solar plexus and claim our independence and power. Parents have dubbed this period "the terrible twos" because it typically becomes a period of frequent power struggles between parents and children, as both try to take control.

In our third year, our caregivers typically adjust to our newfound independence and give us a little more autonomy.

What was it like for you when you were three? Did you get to assert your independence? Did you feel seen by your caregivers?

We all need to feel that we have significance and that we matter. How important is being significant to you now? Be honest.

What have you done in the past to feel important? What accomplishments have you achieved or goals have you attained? Have you sought recognition or other forms of ego-gratification?

This solar plexus need sometimes gets fulfilled in negative ways like workaholism, showing off, or seeking fame or leadership positions for the wrong reasons. It can also show up as an extreme need to be right and, if not curbed, can kill our relationships.

In its most positive form of expression, our need for significance causes us to befriend our ego and pursue meaningful endeavors. It also helps us to value and honor ourselves.

♀ Four-year olds just want to love and be loved, so they hug and cuddle a lot.

AGE 4—HEART: THE NEED TO LOVE AND BE LOVED

♀ The need of our heart chakra is to love and be loved, so we can feel accepted by others and connected them.

This need becomes pretty obvious at age four when we typically enter an easygoing, "cuddly" heart cycle. We have finished exploring the hyper independence of the fiery third chakra cycle, and now we just want to belong and feel a deep, heart connection with our family and friends.

How much love and connection did you experience as a child, especially in your fourth year? How important is love and acceptance to you now? What have you done in the past to gain approval and connection with others? Which parts of

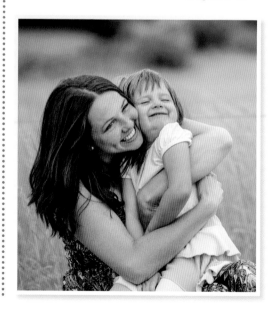

yourself have you hidden or denied in order to feel or appear more loveable? What would you be willing to do or give up in the future to keep another person's affection?

This need can sometimes show up as self-denial where we put our own needs aside in order to do what we think will win another's approval. The benefit of this need is that it motivates us to feel compassion and empathy and to create healthy bonds with others.

The needs of the first four chakras—for safety, variety, significance, and love—are universal needs that all of us actively pursue in one way or another.

In contrast, the needs of the upper chakras do not even seem like "needs" because they are higher level, spiritual desires. Still, as we evolve as a species, these higher chakra needs are growing in importance.

AGE 5–THROAT: THE NEED TO EXPRESS YOUR TRUTH

The need of the throat is to express your personal truth. Through authentic self-expression, we discover who we truly are. This chakra need arises when we are five years old, the time when most of us begin to learn to officially communicate on a social level at school.

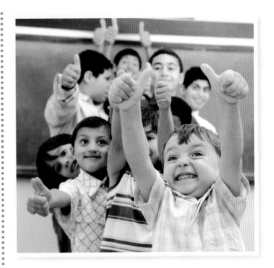

Around age five, we enter school and begin expressing—or hiding—who we really are.

If you were abused in any way in early childhood and were told to keep your abuse secret, you may have serious blockages in this chakra.

People often erroneously believe the throat chakra is more about expression than truth. That's a misunderstanding. Truth is paramount here. Only authentic expression can abide.

The throat chakra is where your deepest life purpose lives, and it will only be revealed through living authentically with every word, every choice, and every action. Your purpose is really just your absolute truth unfolding in every moment, because when you genuinely speak your truth and act on it too, everything false falls away.

How important is living your truth to you? What have you done in the past to live in full integrity with yourself? What have you sacrificed in order for your authentic purpose to unfold? What are you willing to do in the future to facilitate the revelation of your true life purpose? Filling this need fully can show up as a denunciation of conventional living and it can look like you are making radical, illogical choices. Buddha made this kind of radical, fifth chakra choice after the birth of his son, when he left his wife and child behind to follow his path toward enlightenment.

Notice how Buddha's choice may bring up a desire for you to judge. That's normal. As we move farther into the upper chakras, the more misunderstood and judged our choices become, because most people only act from the needs of their lower chakras.

AGE 6—BROW: THE NEED FOR INTUITIVE CONNECTION

♀ The need of the brow chakra is to deeply connect with one's Higher Self. This means attending to and acting on the inner messages that come through your intuition, psychic channels, and spirit guides.

When we are six years old, this manifests as a deep connection to our imagination and fantasy worlds. Ask any six-year-old a simple question and you're bound to get a surprisingly deep answer!

Were you allowed to explore your imagination and express your intuitive experiences (like "imaginary friends") when you were young?

How important is listening to and obeying your Higher Self to you now? What actions have you taken in the past to heed your inner spiritual voice? What would you do in the future to be totally true to your intuitive self and your highest vision?

Fulfilling this need can show up as cultivating unconventional intuitive and psychic talents.

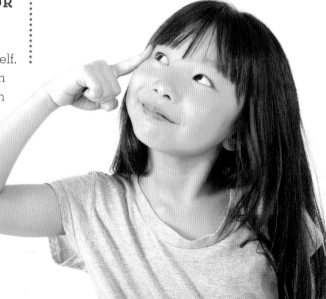

♀ Six-year olds have a vast imagination and ready access to their intuition.

In the past, women were burned at the stake as so-called witches for filling this need. Subconsciously, many of us now hold a fear, at both a soul level and a genetic level, around honoring this part of ourselves. Being aware of this will help you move beyond it.

AGE 7—CROWN: THE NEED FOR ONENESS WITH THE DIVINE

The need of the seventh chakra is to merge with Universal Consciousness and become one with all that is.

We reach a mental and spiritual maturity at seven years of age that allows us to begin to contemplate the concept of being connected to the Divine. Many religions honor a child's capacity to make religious choices at this age. Catholics, for instance, hold communion right around (or soon after) age seven.

What was your spiritual environment around seven years of age? Was it a spiritually open time, or were you told what to believe?

Ask yourself now, how important is complete union with God to you? What have you done in the past to facilitate enlightenment? What would you do in the future to know total union with the Divine?

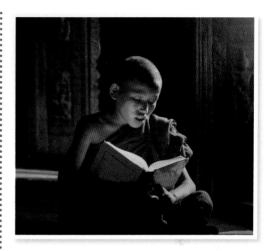

Seven-year-olds want to understand their connection to the Divine.

Fulfilling this need can show up as renunciation of the physical world and complete and utter devotion to God. Monks, priests, and nuns may not totally denounce the physical world, but they usually deny themselves some of life's more desirable pleasures and they definitely commit to God in a deep way.

Absolute enlightenment is a rare thing on this planet. Only a few people in history have attained it in a sustainable way, and that's probably because most people put one or more of their other chakra needs well ahead of this one.

The secondary need of the crown chakra is freedom. We all have a strong need for freedom, because energetically we are pure spirit and anything is possible.

CHAKRA PERSONALITY TYPES AND UNDER- AND OVERACTIVITY

One of the easiest and most convenient ways to assess your chakras is to simply look at your day-to-day habits and your character, since your chakras are the energetic foundation that lead to everything you do and everything you are. Below, I describe the quintessential personality type for each chakra, as well as the common signs of underactivity and overactivity. I share this so you can have a sense of what the energy of each chakra looks like when it is embodied. Keep in mind that when you are very balanced in all your chakras, you will see aspects of yourself in all of these profiles.

In order to give equal time to both genders in this section, I use the masculine pronoun "he" when I describe the masculine (odd-numbered) chakras, and I use the feminine pronoun "she" when I describe the feminine (even-numbered) chakras.

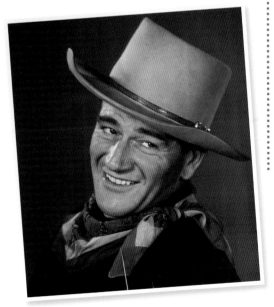

THE ROOT CHAKRA PERSONALITY

A person with strong, balanced root chakra energy is grounded, relaxed, and easy to be around. He may be robust and have a lot of vitality, but it's deep, earthy energy, so he never gives off a frenetic vibe like someone who is overly caffeinated or hyperactive.

- A root chakra person moves steadily, talks less and/or more slowly, makes decisions more cautiously, and likes to plan ahead. He's strong and loyal, and likes things simple and natural.
- He loves family, laughs easily, and has an affable, self-deprecating sense of humor.
- Physically, he's usually sturdy and tends to be stocky rather than light.

John Wayne had the stocky body, slow moves, and humor of the root chakra personality.

- He manifests money and other physical things easily and tends to make everyone around him feel safe and protected.
- **Iconic root chakra person:** Actor John Wayne

ROOT CHAKRA

Underactive	Overactive
Nervous, fearful, anxious	Lazy, bored, tired
Light, hyper, scattered	Heavy, stuck, hoarder
Hates routine, lacks money	Loves routine, overspends,
Has family issues	Ruled by family
Moves homes often	Avoids change

THE SACRAL CHAKRA PERSONALITY

The sacral chakra is the seat of the Divine Feminine. A person who is very open and balanced in this energy center is playful, sensual, and easy-going.

- You want to hang around her, because she's magnetic and enticing.
- She's in touch with her emotions, but doesn't get lost in them, or allow herself to become a drama queen.
- She's extremely creative in the broadest sense of the word, so even if she's not an artist by trade (although she very well may be), she can make a bouquet, cook a meal, or solve a problem in an entertaining or refreshingly new way.

- She's intimacy-oriented, so when you're with her, she makes you feel like you're the only person in the world.
- She's charming and seductive, but try not to count on her too much, because she's too busy flowing, playing, and dancing to pay much attention to schedules and clocks.
- **Iconic sacral chakra person:** Actress Marilyn Monroe

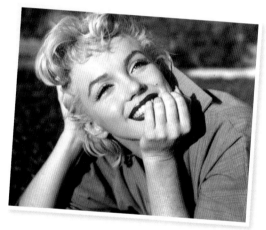

Marilyn Monroe had a seductive, ultra-feminine, sacral chakra personality.

SACRAL CHAKRA

Underactive	Overactive
Overly rational, unresponsive	Irrational, crazy, unstable
Unemotional, not creative	Overly emotional
Intimacy-avoidant	Codependent, neurotic
Frigid, asexual	Promiscuous
Rigid, moves stiffly	Moves well and is flexible

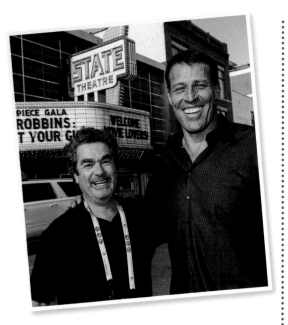

Tony Robbins (right) is a rock star life coach with a confident, fiery solar plexus chakra personality.

- He's dedicated to excellence, so he'll always go the extra mile to make something better. But he he has a fiery temper, and clear personal boundaries, so don't cross him or you might get burned.
- **Iconic solar plexus chakra person:** Life coach Tony Robbins (who has strong feminine energy and empathy)

SOLAR PLEXUS CHAKRA

Underactive	Overactive
Cowardly, timid	Braggart, bully
Passive, or passive-aggressive	Manipulative, controlling
Indecisive, insecure	Know-it-all, egotistical
Scared	Reckless
Procrastinator	Acts too hastily

THE SOLAR PLEXUS PERSONALITY

The strong, balanced solar plexus person is not afraid to be "larger than life," but he doesn't feel that he has to be the center of attention either.

- He's outgoing, interesting, and smart. His mind is quick, his energy is usually high, and he's more than willing to take risks. You'll definitely never be bored around a third chakra guy!
- He's very competitive, but genuinely confident, so if you beat him, he's happy to acknowledge your win.
- Empathy is not his strong suit (unless he has strong feminine energy). It's not that he doesn't care, it's just that his focus is naturally on himself more than anyone else. And somehow, he makes it seem charming.

THE HEART CHAKRA PERSONALITY

Just as you might expect, the heart chakra gal makes love her top priority. Not just romantic love, but familial love, platonic love, and unconditional too.

- She's genuinely balanced in her heart, so she loves herself as much as others, which gives her a strong place from which to share her affections.
- She uses her hands a lot for both hugging others and expressing herself, and carries a natural motherly

energy that makes others feel totally at home.

- She's very open-minded and refreshingly accepting of everybody. This leads to a sort of idealism that sometimes causes her to feel overwhelmed by the way people hurt each other in the world.
- She loves animals as much as people, and she adores nature too.
- She has innate healing abilities and she's so forgiving that it's almost impossible for her to hold a grudge.
- **Iconic heart chakra person:** Diana, Princess of Wales

HEART CHAKRA

Underactive	Overactive
Unsympathetic	Everyone's doormat
Lonely, unsocial	Constant social butterfly
Lacks good relationships	Loses identity in relationships
Unkind, unaware of others	Overly polite, self-conscious
Self-centered	Puts self last

THE THROAT CHAKRA PERSONALITY

The man with a strong throat chakra inspires others with his very essence. He knows who he is, and he doesn't try to be anything else. He's authentic and true, and when he gives you his word, he goes the extra mile to keep it.

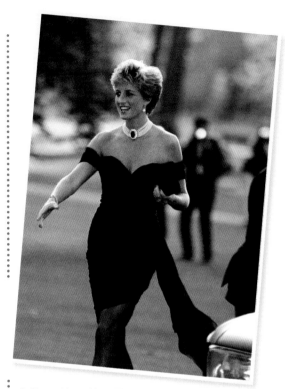

Charitable and loved by millions, Princess Diana had a heart chakra personality.

- He's a great communicator and speaker who can inspire others to action. This is because he has a reason for living, and a big purpose that drives him.
- A natural leader, he generally lives by a clear moral compass, and is a great manifester and visionary. If he chooses to envision and instigate a radical change, there's a good chance he'll succeed at bringing it into the world.
- In most things, he's a man of deep integrity, but he may find it difficult to be romantically faithful.

- He's a dynamic charmer who likes to connect with others so much that monogamy can sometimes be a challenge.
- **Iconic throat chakra person:** Civil rights leader Martin Luther King, Jr.

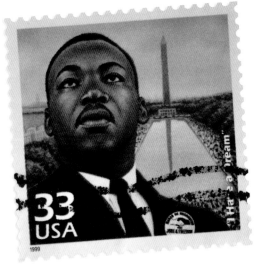

♀ Rev. Martin Luther King, Jr. was an iconic throat chakra personality who had a dream.

THROAT CHAKRA

Underactive	Overactive
Quiet, soft-spoken	Overly talkative, loud
Uncommunicative	Bad listener
Drifts, feels purposeless	Obsessive about causes
Keeps secrets	Shares unsolicited advice and opinions
Pathological liar	Brutally truthful

THE BROW CHAKRA
PERSONALITY

♀ Even as a child, the brow personality's wisdom shines through. She's the kind of gal that everyone goes to for advice, because they trust her perspective.

- She's fair, balanced, and clear. She can look at any situation from numerous perspectives, and can use her intuition to feel into the probable outcomes of different choices.
- There's something deep and mystical and yet so practical and trustworthy about her. If you want her advice, be sure to ask for it, because she's not likely to tell you what she thinks unless you inquire.
- She's so spiritually awake that her entire body is a sensory organ that she can use to feel into any situation, regardless of time or space. She isn't limited by the three dimensions of our physical world.
- Her intuition is so strong that she's incapable of ignoring it, and she's so full of imagination that she's just as happy spending time alone as being with others.
- **Iconic brow chakra person:** Intuitive and author Sonia Choquette

BROW CHAKRA

Underactive	Overactive
Can't visualize	Psychotic visions
Unimaginative	Lives in fantasy world
No intuition	Confused by choices
Uninspired	Overwhelmed by beauty
Cynical	Delusional

THE CROWN CHAKRA
PERSONALITY

As you can imagine, the crown chakra personality is a rare thing, reserved only for those who make spirituality their highest priority and dedicate their life to spiritual, rather than material, pursuits. This crown type is the yogi, guru, or saint who spends a lot of time meditating and connecting directly with source consciousness.

- This personality often wears white to symbolize his connection to the Divine and he typically lives a religious or spiritual life filled with ritual.
- He truly sees the Divine in everyone and everything.
- He loves unconditionally and is nonjudgmental, because he knows that he is one with every person he meets. It is said that Jesus sat with thieves and prostitutes and fully accepted them, because he saw

everyone as a child of God.
- He devotes his entire life to serving others.

CROWN CHAKRA

Underactive	Overactive
Atheist	God complex
Depressed	Manic
Faithless	Spiritual zealot
Too logical	Dizzy or spacy
Materially focused	Financially irresponsible

HOW TO TEST YOUR CHAKRAS WITH WRITTEN TESTS

A necdotal evidence, like the personality characteristics I just shared, can tell you a lot about the state of your chakras. Still, it's always good to do some official testing as well. Written assessments give you a consistent gauge for measuring changes and progress. When clients enroll in my Chakra Abundance course, I have them take an online chakra test before, during, and after they complete the course, so they can actually see their progress. They love watching their scores consistently rise!

Chakra healing creates positive shifts in your life, like more money, better health, more intimacy, etc. And if you tune into your body's subtle energies, you can often feel the ways you have shifted. But due to the fact that your chakras are energetic and intangible, you may sometimes question your conclusions.

It can be very validating to work with something more objective and measurable like a chakra test. One of the best things about written assessments is that they can be repeated to measure consistency or track changes over time.

FINDING RELIABLE WRITTEN TESTS

Written chakra tests are usually pretty easy to take, but unfortunately, there are a lot of inaccurate ones on the internet. This is due to the fact that many so-called "chakra tests" are primarily marketing tools, with their main aim being to collect emails for sales purposes.

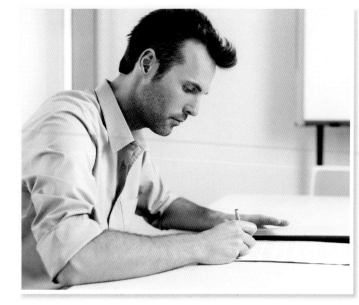

A good written chakra test should have a minimum of seven questions per chakra.

I have taken some of these tests, as have some of my clients, where the results were grossly inaccurate. This is disturbing to me, since many people believe the results and begin doing chakra healings based on their faulty test scores.

My suggestion is to steer clear of any online tests that have fewer than 49 questions (seven for each chakra), because any fewer than seven questions per chakra is too little information for a proper assessment.

I have found one really accurate online test that asks 56 questions and can be taken in several different languages. It genuinely measures your chakras, and I'm happy to report that the creators of the test have never marketed to me. At the time of this writing, you can take this test online at: www.eclecticenergies.com.

Still, you can never be sure if content will stay on the internet, so I have created a series of simple, written tests (one for each chakra) that you can take here and score yourself.

Do them as quickly and honestly as you can. There's nothing to prove, so don't strive for a higher score. You want to aim for accuracy, so you can know the true state of your chakras. Anytime an answer feels neutral, just choose the middle score of 3.

There is one important caveat to written chakra tests that you need to be aware of: they rely on you having an open, active throat chakra. So if, for example, you suspect that your fifth chakra may be particularly underactive, you may want to jump ahead and use the pendulum or applied kinesiology tests, which will be less affected by a fifth chakra weakness.

If you can, take all of the chakra tests quickly in one sitting. When you are finished, check the meaning of your results with the key provided on page 93.

ROOT CHAKRA TEST

Circle the answer that best applies.

1. Can you sit still and be patient?

   1. Not At All
   2. Rarely
   3. Occasionally
   4. Usually
   5. Absolutely

2. Do you generally feel safe?

   1. Not At All
   2. Rarely
   3. Occasionally
   4. Usually
   5. Absolutely

3. Do you feel like you belong on this earth?

   1. Not At All
   2. Rarely
   3. Occasionally
   4. Usually
   5. Absolutely

4. Are you good with money?

   1. Not At All
   2. Rarely
   3. Occasionally
   4. Usually
   5. Absolutely

5. Do you have a good work ethic?

   1. Not At All
   2. Rarely
   3. Occasionally
   4. Usually
   5. Absolutely

6. Are you comfortable in your body?

   1. Not At All
   2. Rarely
   3. Occasionally
   4. Usually
   5. Absolutely

7. Is your home clean and organized?

   1. Not At All
   2. Rarely
   3. Occasionally
   4. Usually
   5. Absolutely

8. Do you order the same dish in your favorite restaurant?

   1. Not At All
   2. Rarely
   3. Occasionally
   4. Usually
   5. Absolutely

9. Do you feel like money comes to you pretty easily?

   1. Not At All
   2. Rarely
   3. Occasionally
   4. Usually
   5. Absolutely

10. When you commit to something, do you stick with it to the end?

    1. Not At All
    2. Rarely
    3. Occasionally
    4. Usually
    5. Absolutely

11. Do you have a strong sense of smell?

    1. Not At All
    2. Rarely
    3. Occasionally
    4. Usually
    5. Absolutely

12. Do you feel grounded and stable?

    1. Not At All
    2. Rarely
    3. Occasionally
    4. Usually
    5. Absolutely

SACRAL CHAKRA TEST

Circle the answer that best applies.

1. Do you find it easy to feel and express your emotions?

   1. Not At All
   2. Rarely
   3. Occasionally
   4. Usually
   5. Absolutely

2. Do you enjoy change and adapt to it easily?

   1. Not At All
   2. Rarely
   3. Occasionally
   4. Usually
   5. Absolutely

3. Are you playful like a kid?

   1. Not At All
   2. Rarely
   3. Occasionally
   4. Usually
   5. Absolutely

4. Do you feel a strong need to be emotionally connected to people?

   1. Not At All
   2. Rarely
   3. Occasionally
   4. Usually
   5. Absolutely

5. Are you able to let go and just "go with the flow?"

   1. Not At All
   2. Rarely
   3. Occasionally
   4. Usually
   5. Absolutely

6. Do you feel comfortable with both intimacy and lust?

   1. Not At All
   2. Rarely
   3. Occasionally
   4. Usually
   5. Absolutely

7. Do you participate in any forms of art?

   1. Not At All
   2. Rarely
   3. Occasionally
   4. Usually
   5. Absolutely

8. Do you feel a need for a lot of variety in your life?

   1. Not At All
   2. Rarely
   3. Occasionally
   4. Usually
   5. Absolutely

9. Are you sensitive to the emotions and moods of others?

   1. Not At All
   2. Rarely
   3. Occasionally
   4. Usually
   5. Absolutely

10. Are you creative?

    1. Not At All
    2. Rarely
    3. Occasionally
    4. Usually
    5. Absolutely

11. Are you an emotional and passionate person?

    1. Not At All
    2. Rarely
    3. Occasionally
    4. Usually
    5. Absolutely

12. Are you able to fully enjoy pleasurable experiences?

    1. Not At All
    2. Rarely
    3. Occasionally
    4. Usually
    5. Absolutely

SOLAR PLEXUS CHAKRA TEST

Circle the answer that best applies.

1. Can you make decisions quickly and definitely?

   1. Not At All
   2. Rarely
   3. Occasionally
   4. Usually
   5. Absolutely

2. In group situations, do you tend to be the one to take control?

   1. Not At All
   2. Rarely
   3. Occasionally
   4. Usually
   5. Absolutely

3. Are you quick-witted?

   1. Not At All
   2. Rarely
   3. Occasionally
   4. Usually
   5. Absolutely

4. Do you believe in yourself completely?

   1. Not At All
   2. Rarely
   3. Occasionally
   4. Usually
   5. Absolutely

5. Do you have a strong will?

   1. Not At All
   2. Rarely
   3. Occasionally
   4. Usually
   5. Absolutely

6. Are you comfortable being the center of attention?

   1. Not At All
   2. Rarely
   3. Occasionally
   4. Usually
   5. Absolutely

7. Are you always aware of what you do and don't like?

   1. Not At All
   2. Rarely
   3. Occasionally
   4. Usually
   5. Absolutely

8. Are you able to be assertive when necessary?

   1. Not At All
   2. Rarely
   3. Occasionally
   4. Usually
   5. Absolutely

9. Are you good at setting and reaching goals?

   1. Not At All
   2. Rarely
   3. Occasionally
   4. Usually
   5. Absolutely

10. Do you often exercise self-restraint?

    1. Not At All
    2. Rarely
    3. Occasionally
    4. Usually
    5. Absolutely

11. Do you feel generally confident, even when trying new things?

    1. Not At All
    2. Rarely
    3. Occasionally
    4. Usually
    5. Absolutely

12. Are you highly motivated (not a procrastinator)?

    1. Not At All
    2. Rarely
    3. Occasionally
    4. Usually
    5. Absolutely

HEART CHAKRA TEST

Circle the answer that best applies.

1. Are you considerate of those around you?

    1. Not At All
    2. Rarely
    3. Occasionally
    4. Usually
    5. Absolutely

2. Are you open and trusting with strangers?

    1. Not At All
    2. Rarely
    3. Occasionally
    4. Usually
    5. Absolutely

3. Do you enjoy sharing with others?

    1. Not At All
    2. Rarely
    3. Occasionally
    4. Usually
    5. Absolutely

4. Do you make cultivating your relationships a high priority?

    1. Not At All
    2. Rarely
    3. Occasionally
    4. Usually
    5. Absolutely

5. Are you able to forgive everyone who wrongs you?

    1. Not At All
    2. Rarely
    3. Occasionally
    4. Usually
    5. Absolutely

6. Are you generous?

    1. Not At All
    2. Rarely
    3. Occasionally
    4. Usually
    5. Absolutely

7. Do you frequently feel gratitude and count your blessings?

    1. Not At All
    2. Rarely
    3. Occasionally
    4. Usually
    5. Absolutely

8. Do you love most people?

    1. Not At All
    2. Rarely
    3. Occasionally
    4. Usually
    5. Absolutely

9. Are you able to easily extend an attitude of compassion to others and yourself?

    1. Not At All
    2. Rarely
    3. Occasionally
    4. Usually
    5. Absolutely

10. Do you make a daily effort to make the people around you feel better?

    1. Not At All
    2. Rarely
    3. Occasionally
    4. Usually
    5. Absolutely

11. Do you hug and cuddle others every day?

    1. Not At All
    2. Rarely
    3. Occasionally
    4. Usually
    5. Absolutely

12. Do you feel elated when something good happens to someone else?

    1. Not At All
    2. Rarely
    3. Occasionally
    4. Usually
    5. Absolutely

THROAT CHAKRA TEST

Circle the answer that best applies.

1. Do you have a clear and audible voice?

    1. Not At All
    2. Rarely
    3. Occasionally
    4. Usually
    5. Absolutely

2. Are you totally honest with everyone (including yourself)?

    1. Not At All
    2. Rarely
    3. Occasionally
    4. Usually
    5. Absolutely

3. Do you have a healthy metabolism (thyroid)?

    1. Not At All
    2. Rarely
    3. Occasionally
    4. Usually
    5. Absolutely

4. Are you interested in communicating with people across the globe?

    1. Not At All
    2. Rarely
    3. Occasionally
    4. Usually
    5. Absolutely

5. Do you balance listening and talking when communicating with others?

    1. Not At All
    2. Rarely
    3. Occasionally
    4. Usually
    5. Absolutely

6. Do you actively engage in some form of self-expression on a regular basis?

    1. Not At All
    2. Rarely
    3. Occasionally
    4. Usually
    5. Absolutely

7. Regardless of what you think your ability is, do you enjoy singing?

    1. Not At All
    2. Rarely
    3. Occasionally
    4. Usually
    5. Absolutely

8. Do you desire to inspire others with your communication?

    1. Not At All
    2. Rarely
    3. Occasionally
    4. Usually
    5. Absolutely

9. Do you keep your promises?

    1. Not At All
    2. Rarely
    3. Occasionally
    4. Usually
    5. Absolutely

10. Do you express your authentic truth even when it's uncomfortable?

    1. Not At All
    2. Rarely
    3. Occasionally
    4. Usually
    5. Absolutely

11. Do you believe the saying, "the truth will set you free?"

    1. Not At All
    2. Rarely
    3. Occasionally
    4. Usually
    5. Absolutely

12. Do you feel you're currently doing your true life's work?

    1. Not At All
    2. Rarely
    3. Occasionally
    4. Usually
    5. Absolutely

BROW CHAKRA TEST

Circle the answer that best applies.

1. Can you visualize easily?

    1. Not At All
    2. Rarely
    3. Occasionally
    4. Usually
    5. Absolutely

2. Do you feel connected to your Higher Self?

    1. Not At All
    2. Rarely
    3. Occasionally
    4. Usually
    5. Absolutely

3. Do you think you'd make a good judge (know what is fair)?

    1. Not At All
    2. Rarely
    3. Occasionally
    4. Usually
    5. Absolutely

4. Do you often know things are going to happen before they do?

    1. Not At All
    2. Rarely
    3. Occasionally
    4. Usually
    5. Absolutely

5. Do you believe in or use any kind of oracles (like cards, pendulums, etc.)?

    1. Not At All
    2. Rarely
    3. Occasionally
    4. Usually
    5. Absolutely

6. Are you good at seeing many different perspectives?

    1. Not At All
    2. Rarely
    3. Occasionally
    4. Usually
    5. Absolutely

7. Do you see a whole lot of beauty in the world?

    1. Not At All
    2. Rarely
    3. Occasionally
    4. Usually
    5. Absolutely

8. Is your intuition strong?

    1. Not At All
    2. Rarely
    3. Occasionally
    4. Usually
    5. Absolutely

9. Have you experienced another realm beyond our physical one?

    1. Not At All
    2. Rarely
    3. Occasionally
    4. Usually
    5. Absolutely

10. Is it easy for you to look within and meditate?

    1. Not At All
    2. Rarely
    3. Occasionally
    4. Usually
    5. Absolutely

11. Are you in touch with your psychic abilities?

    1. Not At All
    2. Rarely
    3. Occasionally
    4. Usually
    5. Absolutely

12. Do you have a vivid imagination?

    1. Not At All
    2. Rarely
    3. Occasionally
    4. Usually
    5. Absolutely

CROWN CHAKRA TEST

Circle the answer that best applies.

1. Do you believe in a Higher Power (God, Source, or Pure Consciousness)?

   1. Not At All
   2. Rarely
   3. Occasionally
   4. Usually
   5. Absolutely

2. Do you enjoy meditating?

   1. Not At All
   2. Rarely
   3. Occasionally
   4. Usually
   5. Absolutely

3. Do you believe that everything happens for a reason?

   1. Not At All
   2. Rarely
   3. Occasionally
   4. Usually
   5. Absolutely

4. Do you believe your soul lives on after physical death?

   1. Not At All
   2. Rarely
   3. Occasionally
   4. Usually
   5. Absolutely

5. Do you have some kind of regular, spiritual practice?

   1. Not At All
   2. Rarely
   3. Occasionally
   4. Usually
   5. Absolutely

6. Are you able to live fully in the now (and not be pulled into the future or past)?

   1. Not At All
   2. Rarely
   3. Occasionally
   4. Usually
   5. Absolutely

7. Do you believe there is order behind everything in the universe?

   1. Not At All
   2. Rarely
   3. Occasionally
   4. Usually
   5. Absolutely

8. Do you regularly engage in spiritual rituals of any kind?

   1. Not At All
   2. Rarely
   3. Occasionally
   4. Usually
   5. Absolutely

9. Do you believe the saying, "We are all one"?

   1. Not At All
   2. Rarely
   3. Occasionally
   4. Usually
   5. Absolutely

10. Do you believe synchronicities are a sign from above?

    1. Not At All
    2. Rarely
    3. Occasionally
    4. Usually
    5. Absolutely

11. Do you believe your essence lives beyond time and space?

    1. Not At All
    2. Rarely
    3. Occasionally
    4. Usually
    5. Absolutely

12. Do you pray or otherwise communicate with a higher power?

    1. Not At All
    2. Rarely
    3. Occasionally
    4. Usually
    5. Absolutely

YOUR CHAKRA TEST RESULTS

Add up the combined points (the numbers circled) for each chakra and consult the key below.

52–60 POINTS: OVERACTIVE

This chakra is so open and strong that it may be causing an imbalance in your energy field, and issues in the areas of life that relate to your other chakras. If, however, all your chakras are "overactive," you probably just have a super-boosted, balanced energy field.

44–51 POINTS: OPEN & BALANCED

This chakra is open in a healthy way that is optimal for a balanced energy field.

35–43 POINTS: SLIGHTLY UNDERACTIVE

This chakra is currently a little underactive for good balance, especially if the other chakras in your field are open and balanced, or overactive.

26–34 POINTS: VERY UNDERACTIVE

This chakra is currently very underactive, and could use your loving attention and regular healing practices, such as those outlined in chapter three.

25 POINTS OR LESS: BLOCKED

This chakra is currently extremely underactive and indicates there is probably a serious blockage at any or all of these levels: mental, emotional, and physical.

Focus your attention on the chakras with the lowest scores until you see a marked improvement.

GRAPH YOUR CHAKRA RESULTS

If you want to see the big picture of your chakra results, create a graph like the one below. Put the possible scores in increments of five on the y axis and the seven chakras on the x axis. Then, use colored pens or crayons to plot your chakra scores. This gives you a great visual representation of the relationship between your chakras.

This graph shows Upper Chakra Dominance and a need for grounding.

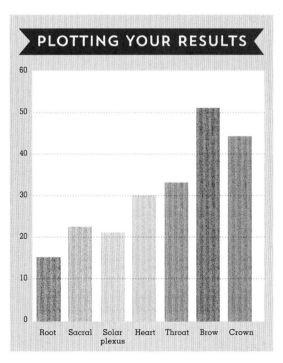

PLOTTING YOUR RESULTS

USING A PENDULUM TO TEST THE CHAKRAS

A pendulum is a great tool for directly observing the energetic spin of the chakras. You simply dangle it over each chakra, allowing it to be moved by the vortex energy, and note the different qualities of the movement like rotation size, direction, and shape. Each of these things tells you something about the state of the chakra you're assessing at any given time. Unfortunately, this is not a good method for assessing your own chakras, so it should be reserved for when you can work with a partner.

When you have found someone with whom you want to perform a pendulum chakra assessment, make sure to do these three things before you begin:

1. CHOOSE A GOOD PENDULUM

⚲ Whenever you assess or gauge something (particularly something intangible like a chakra), you need to make sure your measuring tool is reliable and consistent.

When it comes to the chakras, a basic, conical wood pendulum is the most neutral and therefore most reliable one you can use. Other types of pendulums like those made of metal or gemstones might not remain consistent across all seven chakras. Some gemstone pendulums may resonate more with certain chakras over others, and some high-frequency stones like selenite, kyanite, or aurora quartz may magnify the energy of *all* the chakras.

A nice, light wood, like beechwood, is a good material for a chakra pendulum.

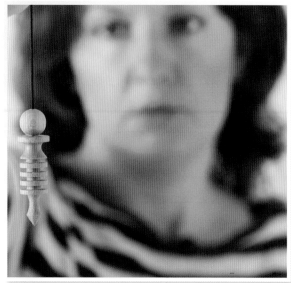

⚲ Wooden pendulums are the best for chakra work because, unlike metal or gemstones, wood is neutral.

Additionally, be sure to choose a pendulum that is symmetrical. That way, if it makes asymmetrical movements during a reading, you will know they are being caused by the chakra's energy, and not by any asymmetry in the pendulum itself.

2. ACCLIMATE YOUR PENDULUM TO YOUR OWN ENERGY FIELD

When you assess the chakras of another person with a pendulum, your personal energy can affect the results. For this reason, it's important that you acclimate your pendulum to your own chakras first, and reduce any effect your energy might have on someone else's reading.

Likewise, if someone is going to assess your chakras, make sure they have first acclimated their pendulum to their energy field as well.

The simplest way to acclimate a pendulum is to carry it on your body for a minimum of three days.

It can also be helpful to do a small ritual when you first get it. Hold it in your cupped hands and say this prayer (or something similar):

"I honor and bless this pendulum for the healing and information it will impart. I invite it to calibrate to my energy field now, so that from this time forward, it only responds to and measures the energy of others."

3. CLEAR YOUR MIND AND SET THE INTENTION TO BE A CHANNEL OF HEALING

Your thoughts and intentions literally move energy, so it's very important that you clear you mind before assessing someone's chakras. One thing that helps to get your personal thoughts out of the way is to say a little prayer.

Try this one:
"I let go of any preconceptions or ideas I might have about [their name]'s chakras, and invite pure truth to come through me and this pendulum for the highest purpose of clarity and healing."

You also want to quietly repeat this statement three times:
"Just be blank."

Try it. You'll be amazed at how well it works!

Once you have completed these three things, you are ready to perform a chakra reading using your pendulum by following the steps described on the following page.

HOW TO DIRECTLY ASSESS YOUR CHAKRAS WITH A PENDULUM

1. Have the person you are assessing lie down on her back, close her eyes, and relax.

2. Start at either her root chakra or crown, and work your way up or down her body through the seven chakras. For this example, we'll start at the root.

3. Using the hand that feels intuitively right to you, hold the pendulum with it draped over the side of your index finger so that your palm chakra won't affect the reading. If you pinch it between your thumb and index finger and dangle it, your own palm chakra is directly facing the pendulum and can greatly affect its spin.

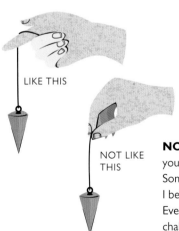

LIKE THIS

NOT LIKE THIS

4. Dangle the pendulum 2–3 inches (2.5–7.6 cm) above the body in the area of the root chakra, just below the groin. Start far enough down the body that you can be sure not miss the root chakra and then slowly and steadily move the pendulum up the body until it gets swept into the vortex of the root chakra. Usually, you will feel a very gentle pulling sensation as you get near it, and you simply follow it.

5. Once the pendulum is in the vortex of the chakra, observe its movement. Note the size, shape, and direction of the motion and use the Chakra Pendulum Key (see facing page) to interpret what it means.

6. Do the same with all the other chakras, recording the results, and interpreting what they mean using the key.

7. When you're done with assessing all the chakras, say a prayer of thanks for receiving the information and respectfully put away your pendulum.

NOTE: Once you know which chakras need healing, you can engage in your preferred form of healing. Some people like to use the pendulum to heal, but I believe there are many stronger forms of therapy. Even just using your own hand—with its powerful palm chakra—is preferable. So unless the pendulum resonates deeply with you as a healing tool, I advise using it only for assessment.

CHAKRA PENDULUM KEY

Below you will find the most common interpretations for pendulum movements when assessing a chakra. But energy can be idiosyncratic, so be sure to experiment with your pendulum to see what's true for you.

DIRECTION

- **Clockwise**—the chakra is open and functioning optimally.
- **Counterclockwise**—the chakra is blocked in a psychodynamic way. Deep beliefs are causing opposition to the normal spin.

SHAPE

- **Circular**—the chakra is open and has good masculine–feminine balance.
- **Elliptical**—the chakra is imbalanced toward the masculine or feminine. If the top (crown side) of the elliptical motion points to the right, the chakra carries more masculine energy. If the top of the elliptical points to the left, the chakra has more feminine energy.

SIZE

Chakras can be many different sizes and still be functional and acceptable. The most important thing is how the chakras relate to each other. You want to look for, and encourage, consistent size across all the chakras, so the whole field is balanced. The sizes here only apply if the pendulum is close to the body (about 2–3 inches [2.5–7.6 cm] above it), because the chakra vortices extend outward and the diameter widens as you go farther out.

- **Small** (1 inch [2.5 cm] or less diameter)—the chakra is unusually closed/underactive.
- **Middle** ($1^{1}/_{2}$–4 inches [3.8–10 cm] diameter)—in the open range.
- **Large** (over $4^{1}/_{2}$ inches [11.4 cm] diameter)—the chakra is abnormally open/overactive (but can be good, if all are this size).

These measurements are all relational. Their meanings vary according to how far away from the body you measure. Also, keep in mind that if a chakra is larger than normal, it's not "overactive" if the other chakras are equally expanded.

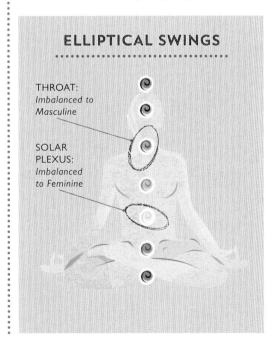

ELLIPTICAL SWINGS

THROAT:
Imbalanced to Masculine

SOLAR PLEXUS:
Imbalanced to Feminine

HOW TO INDIRECTLY ASSESS YOUR CHAKRAS USING A PENDULUM

Since you can't do a good direct assessment of your own chakras with a pendulum, you may want to do an indirect pendulum reading. This process is called pendulum dowsing, and it entails using the pendulum to read your chakras (or answer other spiritual questions) by proxy.

Pendulum dowsing is an art that deserves a whole chapter of its own, so this section is just a primer. If it intrigues you, I advise you to study it further.

Before you start doing a chakra dowsing reading, do the preparatory steps mentioned on page 94: Choose a good pendulum, acclimate it to your energy field, and clear your mind. Then do the following:

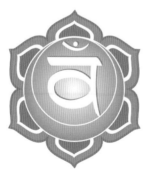

1. Hold the pendulum draped over your index finger (as described on page 96) so that your palm chakras don't affect its spin.

2. Ask the pendulum a question with an obvious "yes" answer, like, "Is my name [your name here]?" The pendulum's response becomes your indicator for "yes." If it isn't clear, you can ask a second obvious "yes" question to see if it is replicated. Ask as many questions as you need to determine your "yes" indicator.

3. Once your "yes" response has been clearly identified, ask an obvious "no" question like, "Am I five years old?" The pendulum's response becomes your indicator for "no." Again, if it isn't clear, you can ask a second obvious "no" question to see if it is replicated, and repeat as needed to determine your "no" indicator.

4. Once you have clear "yes" and "no" indicators, you can ask the pendulum any yes or no question about your chakras that you'd like and see which indicator you get. The simplest method is to go through each chakra and ask if it is healthy and open. In this way, you can assess your entire chakra system.

PENDULUM ASSESSMENT USING
A CHAKRA CHART

Another type of pendulum dowsing you can do involves using a chakra chart. Here are the steps:

1. Copy or create a chart like the one below.

2. Lay it flat and hold your pendulum over the convergence point (at the arrow point).

3. Ask to be shown the chakra that most needs healing.

4. Observe where the pendulum goes. When it swings in a particular chakra zone, that chakra needs healing.

5. Ask about the next chakra that most needs healing, and so on, until you no longer get an indication from the pendulum that any chakras need healing.

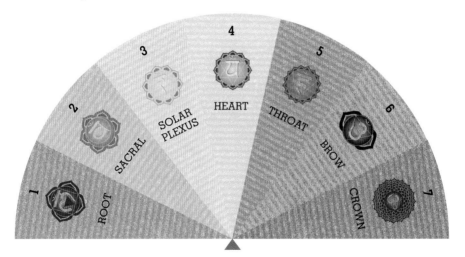

Regardless of which pendulum method you choose to use, make sure you always keep your arm steady, but relaxed. If you tense up, you restrict the energy flow and the pendulum can't receive the information it needs to move accurately.

USING APPLIED KINESIOLOGY TO ASSESS THE CHAKRAS

Applied kinesiology, which is also known as muscle testing, is a great way to directly access your body's wisdom without your thoughts or judgments getting in the way. The human body functions best when it's in full integrity, so any time we state something that is untrue, we get weaker. This is why lie detectors work. They measure the stress our body goes into when we lie.

Muscle testing works in a similar way, but without any need for a high-tech machine. When we do applied kinesiology, we are using the strength (or weakness) of our body to tell us whether a statement is true.

The premise is very simple: When we say a true statement, our muscles react with integrity and strength, and when we tell a lie, our muscles weaken and give way.

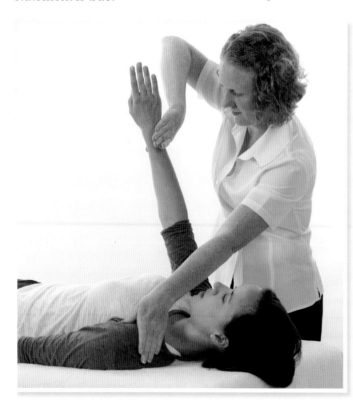

Applied kinesiology is a simple and powerful way to get accurate "yes" or "no" answers about the state of your chakras. Doing it requires a certain level of kinesthetic sensitivity, so you may have to practice a bit to get a feel for it. Still, if you approach it with intellectual curiosity and do it fairly regularly, you'll find that it's an amazingly accurate way to assess your chakras (or any other area of your life).

If a person is injured or ill, you can do applied kinesiology lying down.

USING APPLIED KINESIOLOGY TO ASSESS YOUR OWN CHAKRAS

You can muscle test your own chakras as well. Here are the steps:

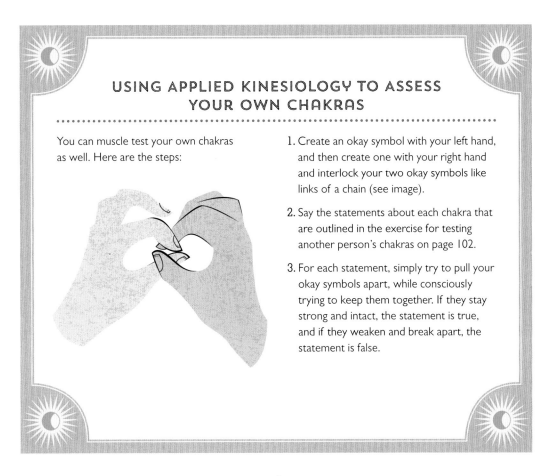

1. Create an okay symbol with your left hand, and then create one with your right hand and interlock your two okay symbols like links of a chain (see image).

2. Say the statements about each chakra that are outlined in the exercise for testing another person's chakras on page 102.

3. For each statement, simply try to pull your okay symbols apart, while consciously trying to keep them together. If they stay strong and intact, the statement is true, and if they weaken and break apart, the statement is false.

QUICK ASSESSMENT TECHNIQUE

If you want to do a quick, non-verbal assessment to discover which chakras need healing, you can simply have the person you're testing put their right hand over each chakra and muscle test each one. The healthy and open chakras will test strong and the blocked or underactive chakras will test weak and collapse.

Here are the areas for hand placement:

- **Root**—lowest part of groin
- **Sacral Chakra**—right under navel
- **Solar Plexus Chakra**—over solar plexus, where the ribs part
- **Heart Chakra**—middle of the chest
- **Throat Chakra**—middle of the throat
- **Brow Chakra**—above and between the eyebrows
- **Crown Chakra**—at the very top of the head

MUSCLE TESTING TO ASSESS
ANOTHER PERSON'S CHAKRAS

To measure the state of someone's chakras with applied kinesiology, follow these simple steps.

1. Have them stand up (or sit upright in a chair) and stand right behind them.

2. Ask them to straighten their left arm and point it directly left at shoulder height with their palm down.

3. Put your right hand on their right shoulder for anchoring stability, place two or three fingers of your left hand on top of their hand near their wrist and ask them to resist fully whenever you push down.

5. Have them say an obviously true statement like, *"I am (their name)."* As

soon as they say it, press down firmly on their left hand. It should be steady and resistant. Note the firmness. This is their indicator that a statement is true.

6. Next, have them say an obviously false statement like, *"I am one year old,"* and press down on their left hand with the same amount of pressure you used before. It should weaken and collapse. This is their indicator that a statement is false.

7. Now that you know what their bodily response is for a true and false statement, you can assess the chakras.

8. Simply have the person go through each one of their seven chakras and say, *"My ___ chakra is healthy and open."* If it tests as true, then have them move onto the next chakra. If it tests as false, then you want to discover if the chakra is under- or overactive. Have them say, *"My ___ chakra is underactive."* If it tests as true, then move onto the next chakra. If it tests as false, then have them say, *"My ___ chakra is overactive."*

9. Through this process, you will be able to discover which chakras are healthy and open and which ones are either under- or overactive.

CHAKRA-RELATED ISSUES AND DISEASES

Because it takes quite a while for energy to manifest in the physical world, diseases tell us which chakras have been out of balance for a while. In other words, illnesses typically show us where the chronic chakra imbalances are. In this section, I give you a list of the common illnesses and diseases related to each chakra, but no list can be exhaustive, so I'm going to show you how to determine which issues are generally associated with each chakra.

It's actually a surprisingly logical process. You simply ask yourself these questions:

1. WHERE IS THE DISEASE LOCATED?

If an illness shows up in a specific area, it is almost always related to the chakra that governs that area of the body.

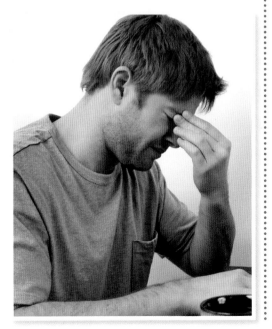

2. IS THE ILLNESS RELATED TO A PARTICULAR ENDOCRINE GLAND?

As described in chapter one, each chakra is associated with a specific endocrine gland. So, if an endocrine gland is related to a particular disease, then the chakra for that gland is probably associated with the disease as well.

When we look at the diseases and illnesses that are typically associated with each chakra, be aware that you may see opposite issues in the same chakra, like anorexia and obesity in the root chakra. This is because one illness signifies that the person is underactive in the chakra, and the other illness signifies that the individual is overactive.

♀ All illnesses begin at the energy level and are rooted in one or more of the chakras.

Additionally, because our beliefs feed our chakras, a person can be overactive in one aspect of a chakra, while being underactive in another.

For instance, if a woman is really insecure, the self-esteem aspect of her third chakra may be very underactive, and yet the action-taking part of her third chakra could be really overactive, because she's constantly trying to prove her worth through her actions and accomplishments. Or, if a man was sexually abused as a child, the emotional part of his sacral chakra could be shut down, while the sexual part could be overactive.

ADDICTIONS

Addictions are a form of illness that tell us a lot about our chakras. All addictions are based in the root chakra, the energy center of memory and repetition, but the nature of the addiction—food, drugs, sex, etc.—often involves an additional chakra influence. You may notice that the most common addictions only apply to the lower (bodily) chakras, because that's where the biggest physiological traps lie. Still, a person could have upper chakra-oriented addictions like over-using witchcraft (brow chakra) or obsessively meditating (crown chakra).

CHAKRA ASSOCIATIONS FOR COMMON ADDICTIONS

Alcohol	overactive root, overactive solar plexus
Cocaine or crack	overactive root, underactive solar plexus
Coffee	underactive root, underactive solar plexus
Food	overactive root
Gambling	overactive root, underactive solar plexus
Marijuana	overactive root, underactive or overactive sacral
Nicotine	overactive root, underactive or overactive solar plexus
Sex	overactive root, overactive sacral, underactive heart
Shopping	overactive root
Work	overactive root, underactive or overactive solar plexus

ROOT CHAKRA ISSUES

♀ Any illness or injury that is located in the area from the feet up to the tailbone is most likely related to the root chakra. Also, any of these:

- Diseases of the intestines, colon, anus, rectum, or any issue related to elimination.
- The 3 Bs—Any issue associated with bones, bowels, or blood.
- Skin problems from eczema to leprosy.
- For men, diseases of the testes, like prostate cancer or any kind of infertility.
- All addictions are associated with the root chakra, because they are about the body's memory, homeostasis, and repetition, which are all qualities of the first chakra.

SACRAL CHAKRA ISSUES

♀ The sacral chakra governs the pelvic bowl and lower back area. Here are the illnesses that are associated with it:

- Issues involving the ovaries, like female reproduction or hormonal problems, menstrual irregularities, PMS, and other forms of chronic emotional swings.
- Urinary or bladder problems, or dehydration (since the sacral chakra relates to the water element).
- STDs (sexually transmitted diseases).
- Scoliosis, because when there is a weak root chakra combined with too much second chakra energy, our bones literally curve.

♀ Menstrual cramps and other women's issues are related to the sacral chakra.

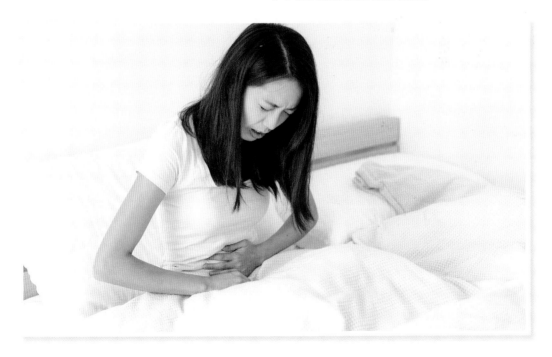

SOLAR PLEXUS CHAKRA ISSUES

The solar plexus chakra is associated with any illness related to the digestive or filtering organs like the stomach, liver, pancreas, gallbladder, spleen, and kidneys, as well as these:

- Food allergies, glucose imbalances, gout, gastritis, or ulcers.
- Adrenal problems or chronic fatigue.
- Insomnia or sleep issues (due to too much solar plexus, "sun" energy).
- Male impotence, because the penis, and its ability to become erect, is associated with the fiery, goal-oriented energy of the solar plexus chakra.

HEART CHAKRA ISSUES

The most obvious problems here are any that are associated with the heart or breasts such as heart attacks, arrhythmias, or breast cancer. Plus, the following issues:

- Breath-oriented diseases such as the "3 As"—asthma, allergies, and apnea—as well as bronchitis.
- Colds, flus, or pneumonia.
- Failure to thrive (when babies aren't loved and hugged).
- Thymus or auto-immune problems such as lupus.
- Carpel tunnel syndrome and tendinitis in the elbow, because heart energy runs down the arms. If these issues show up on the right side of the body, they are related to a weakness in the masculine heart (giving or showing love), and if they are on the left side of the body, they are associated with weakness in the feminine heart chakra (receiving love).

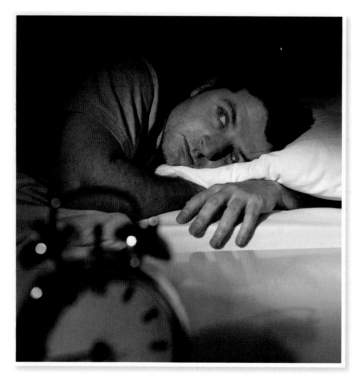

Insomnia is due to an underactive first chakra and overactive third, sixth, and seventh chakras.

THROAT CHAKRA ISSUES

The throat chakra governs the area from the base of the throat up to the ears, so the following illnesses are related to it:

- Diseases of the throat, tonsils, and larynx like strep throat, tonsillitis, and laryngitis.
- Jaw issues like TMJ (lockjaw).
- Ear problems like infections and tinnitus.
- Thyroid problems such as hyperthyroidism (overactive), hypothyroidism (underactive), Graves' disease, and Hashimoto's disease.

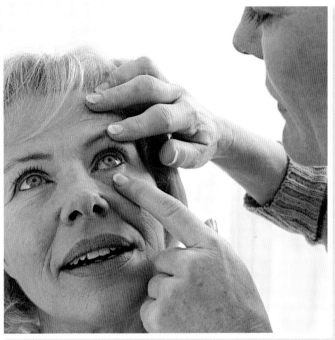

Eye diseases and vision problems are related to the brow chakra.

BROW CHAKRA ISSUES

The third eye governs our head from the sinuses up. Here are the diseases related to it:

- Vision problems like conjunctivitis, glaucoma, or cataracts.
- Certain brain problems like migraines and dyslexia.
- Pineal gland issues like seasonal affective disorder (SAD) or bad jetlag.
- Sinusitis and chronic rhinitis.

CROWN CHAKRA ISSUES

The crown chakra's domain is mostly the nervous system and brain, so it's related to the following:

- Disorders or diseases that are associated with delusional or disrupted brain states like dizziness, bipolar, and schizophrenia.
- Neurological problems like Parkinson's disease, multiple sclerosis, or epilepsy.
- Brain diseases like cancer, meningitis, or encephalitis.
- Chronic depression is usually a sign of an underactive crown chakra.

CHAKRA-RELATED ILLNESSES AND DISEASES

Note: This table is not in any way intended to be medically prescriptive. It is provided for anecdotal purposes only. If you have any symptoms of any illness or disease, please seek guidance from a health care professional.

KEY:

O = Overactive

U = Underactive

E = Either Overactive or Underactive

+ = Other chakras involved in the issue:

1st = Root Chakra

2nd = Sacral Chakra

3rd = Solar Plexus Chakra

4th = Heart Chakra

5th = Throat Chakra

6th = Brow Chakra

7th = Crown Chakra

ROOT CHAKRA

- Addictions (O)
- Anemia (U)
- Anorexia (U)
- Athlete's foot (O)
- Arthritis (U)
- Bipolar (O) + 3rd (U), 7th (O)
- Blood pressure: High (O), Low (U)
- Chronic fatigue (O) + 3rd (U)
- Colitis (O)
- Constipation (U)
- Crohn's disease (O) + 3rd (O)
- Depression (O) + 7th (U)
- Diarrhea or overactive bowels (O) + 2nd (O)
- Eczema (O)
- Edema (O)
- Gallstones (O) + 3rd (O)
- Gout (O) + 3rd (O)
- Hemorrhoids (U)
- Hives (O) + chakra break out area (O)
- Irritable bowel syndrome (O) + 3rd (U)
- Insomnia (U) + 3rd (O), 6th (O), 7th (O)
- Kidney stones (O) + 3rd (O)
- Obesity (O) + 3rd (U)
- OCD (O) + 7th (U)
- Sciatica (E)
- Scoliosis (U) + 2nd (O)
- Shingles (O)
- Sleep apnea (O) + 4th (U)
- Sterility [male] (U)

SACRAL CHAKRA

- Bladder problems (O)
- Dehydration (U)
- Endometriosis (O)
- Herpes (O)
- Hip problems (E)
- Infertility [female] (U)
- Impotence (U) + 3rd (U)
- Menstrual problems (E)
- PMS (O) + 3rd (O)
- Scoliosis (O) + 1st (U)
- Sexual frigidity (U)
- STDs (O)
- Urinary infections (O)

SOLAR PLEXUS CHAKRA

- Abdominal hernia (O)
- Bipolar (U) + 1st (O), 7th (O)
- Breast cancer (U) + 4th (O)
- Chronic fatigue (U) + 1st (O)
- Crohn's disease (O) + 1st (O)
- Diabetes (U)
- Dyslexia (U) + 6th (O)
- Food allergies (U)
- Gallstones (O) + 1st (O)
- Gastritis (O)
- Gout (O) + 1st (O)
- Hepatitis (E)
- Hypoglycemia (U)
- Impotence (U) + 2nd (U)
- Indigestion of all kinds (E)
- Insomnia (O) + 1st (U) , 6th (O), 7th (O)
- Irritable bowel syndrome (U) + 1st (O)
- Jaundice (U)
- Kidney stones (O) + 1st (O)
- Liver disease (E)
- Nausea (E)
- Obesity (U) + 1st (O)
- Pancreatitis (O)
- PMS (O) + 2nd (O)
- Stuttering (U) + 5th (U)
- Tourette syndrome (O) + 5th (U)
- Ulcers (O)

HEART CHAKRA

- Allergies (non-food) (O)
- Asthma (U)
- Breast cancer (O) + 3rd (U)
- Bronchitis (U) + 5th (U)
- Carpal tunnel syndrome (O)
- Colds (U)
- Emphysema (U)
- Cardiovascular diseases (E)
- Heart arrhythmia (E)
- Lupus (U)
- Pneumonia (U)
- Sleep apnea (U) + 1st (O)
- Tendonitis in arms or hands (O)

THROAT CHAKRA

- Bronchitis (U) + 4th (U)
- Ear infections (E)
- Goiter (O)
- Hearing problems (E)
- Hyperthyroidism (O)
- Hypothyroidism (U)
- Laryngitis (U)
- Stuttering (U) + 3rd (U)
- Teeth and gum issues (E)
- Tinnitus (U)
- TMJ/Lockjaw (U)
- Tonsillitis (O)
- Tourette syndrome (U) + 3rd (O)

BROW CHAKRA

- Cataracts (O)
- Conjunctivitis (O)
- Dizziness (O) + 7th
- Dyslexia (O) + 3rd (U)
- Insomnia (O) + 1st (U), 3rd (O), 7th (O)
- Glaucoma (O)
- Migraines (O)
- Seasonal Affective Disorder (SAD) (O)
- Sinus problems (E)
- Vision problems (E)

CROWN CHAKRA

- Alzheimer's (O)
- Bipolar (O), + 1st (O), 3rd (U)
- Brain cancer (O)
- Depression (U) + 1st (O)
- Dizziness (O)
- Encephalitis (O)
- Epilepsy (O)
- Insomnia (O) + 1st (U), 3rd (O), 6th (O)
- Meningitis (O)
- Multiple sclerosis (U)
- OCD (U) + 1st (O)
- Parkinson's disease (U)
- Schizophrenia (O)
- Stroke (O)

CHAKRA-RELATED "ACCIDENTS"

After years of doing chakra work with clients, I have come to realize that our accidents are often tied to a particular chakra. If you subscribe to the belief that accidents happen "to" you, this concept may be hard to grasp, so allow me to explain. In truth, we are not separate from anything, but are living and moving in a collective energy field that is constantly unified.

For this reason, we not only manifest diseases and illnesses from the energies that are within us, but we have accidents that are either an expression of the energies within us, or a magnetized reaction to the energies within us. Let me share a couple of examples, one from my own life and one from a client.

HOW ACCIDENTS MATCH OUR CHAKRA ENERGY

Years ago before I started doing chakra healing, I had a private yoga client, Ted, who was going through a difficult divorce. Though he tried hard not to show it, I could tell his heart chakra was in distress. His shoulders began to curl forward a little more than usual, and his left shoulder—which is related to his feminine heart, female partner, and receiving love—ached most of the time. In our yoga sessions, we created some temporary shifts that caused the pain to subside for a while, but that nasty shoulder issue kept popping back up (which is one of the reasons I started doing energy healing, because all physical issues begin in our chakras).

When Ted dislocated his left shoulder while skiing, it seemed symbolically perfect. He had hurt himself exactly where he had been experiencing so much grief (in the feminine side of his heart chakra) and the concept of "dislocation" matched his feeling about his divorce, as he was living in a temporary rental away from his young son.

A similar situation happened in my life. Some years ago, I had self-diagnosed a serious root chakra issue, so I was doing a lot of practices to boost my first chakra. I took my son roller skating, and although I hadn't been on roller skates for at least 25 years, I thought I could handle skating backward. A woman inadvertently put her skate out into my path and I fell hard on my tailbone. Although it was an "accident," it hardly seemed random that I fell right in the area where I most needed chakra activation.

My roller-skating injury actually activated a deep root chakra healing.

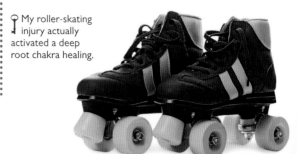

⚡ A shoulder or arm injury could be a sign of heart chakra imbalance.

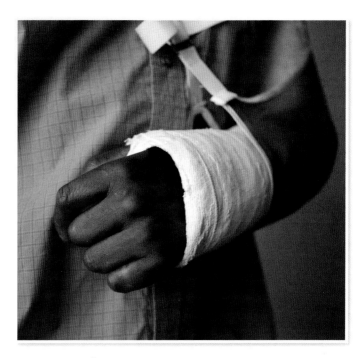

CHAKRA ACTIVATION THROUGH INJURY

From my experience in working with the chakras, I not only believe that our accidents typically point to our biggest chakra weaknesses, but more importantly, they often activate us through injury. What better way to open an energy center than a break, sprain, or painful smack right on it?

Anytime you experience an illness or an injury, ask yourself: What might this be showing me about my chakras? Look at the chakra area in which it takes place, the endocrine glands (if any) involved, and consult the table on pages 108 and 109. When you dive into the chakra influences behind your issues, illnesses, and accidents, you can turn a challenging or painful situation into a goldmine of self-understanding and personal growth.

KEYNOTE

Most people call chakra healing an "alternative" therapy, but it's actually better to consider it an adjunct therapy, since it works very well alongside the more traditional, allopathic options. This information on the relationship between chakras and illnesses is provided for self-exploration only and should not be considered medical advice. If you are suffering from any health issues, seek professional medical assistance.

THE THREE MAIN CHAKRA TYPES

Not only can we assess each individual chakra, but it's also very helpful to look at the big picture of our entire chakra system. Over many years of doing yoga and chakra work with my clients, I've discovered that most of us tend to reside more in one area of our energy field over the others. Over time, I came to identify three key patterns I call the main chakra types.

As I describe them here, feel into each one and see if it applies to you, because once you figure out what type (or hybrid) you are, it's easier to choose the right activities that will bring you more chakra balance and personal expansion.

Keep in mind that this typology is necessarily generalized and only a temporary assessment. Still, it's useful to identify the unhealthy or unhelpful patterns that come from your beliefs, heredity, and habits, so you can find a gateway to embodying more of your full, energetic potential.

The three main chakra types are: Upper Chakra Dominant (Upper), Lower Chakra Dominant (Lower), and Split.

An Upper lives more in their upper chakras, a Lower lives primarily in their lower chakras, and a Split bounces back and forth between the upper and lower chakra realms. This is due to the fact that Splits tend to avoid the solar plexus chakra that creates integrity between the two.

THE UPPER CHAKRA DOMINANT TYPE

Uppers live more in the spiritual realm. They tend to be more connected to their intuition, psychic abilities, and higher guides. These people are often labeled "highly sensitive," because they are very aware of energy and can feel it as surely as physical touch. For this reason, they can get lost or overwhelmed by the energy of others.

Because they live mostly in the upper part of their energy field, they are also farther away from the safe energies of the root chakra, which can make them feel and act scattered and ungrounded. And since energy moves more quickly in the upper chakras, they tend to talk and move faster than others.

Uppers typically hold beliefs—either consciously or subconsciously—that being fully in their body is unsafe or can compromise their spiritual integrity. They tend to judge lower chakra things like wealth, sexuality, and power, but due to their deep identification with spirituality, they typically won't admit they are judging these things. Because of this, Uppers usually struggle with finances and the day-to-day logistics of life.

They can be commitment-phobic as well, because the first chakra is about being rooted and staying in place, while the upper chakras are about being able to move around quickly and freely. This means Uppers tend to move and change things in their life like their home, job, and relationships quite frequently.

Because they aren't very grounded, Uppers usually feel unsafe, and this lack of security causes them to feel anxious much of the time.

A great metaphor for the Upper is the untethered helium balloon. It has a lot of

The Upper Chakra Dominant type is like an untethered balloon, free but ungrounded.

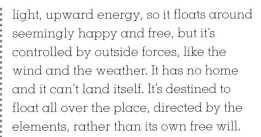

light, upward energy, so it floats around seemingly happy and free, but it's controlled by outside forces, like the wind and the weather. It has no home and it can't land itself. It's destined to float all over the place, directed by the elements, rather than its own free will.

THE LOWER CHAKRA DOMINANT TYPE

As you might expect, Lowers are basically the energetic opposite of Uppers. They are grounded in the physical world and handle it quite well. In marked contrast to the Uppers who tend to reflect the frenetic freedom of unlimited crown energy, Lowers embody the stability, consistency, and slower pace of the root.

They enjoy the material world and are generally good at manifesting things. Basically, they are comfortable in their skin, and they are close with their tribe, the friends and family that make up their extended social circle.

Lowers are loyal, longstanding creatures of habit who typically don't like change, especially if it comes suddenly or chaotically. When they go to their favorite restaurant, they usually prefer to order their tried-and-true dish, instead of trying something new.

Lowers can get caught in a rut, or even get totally stuck, in complete contrast to

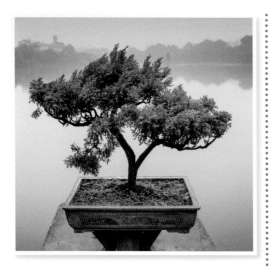

The Lower Chakra Dominant type is like an over-pruned tree—rooted, but not free to grow.

Uppers who tend to make so many changes that their lives lack continuity, order, and stability.

Whereas the Uppers usually fear going down into the embodied zone of the lower chakras, the Lowers actually aspire to go into the upper chakras. But because they're so well connected to the physical realm, it can be very challenging for them to get beyond their day-to-day worldly concerns.

For this reason, Lowers rarely feel anxiety like the Uppers. Instead, they tend to experience its opposite, depression.

A good metaphor for the Lower is the over-pruned tree. It has really good roots and is healthy and stable, but it can't grow fully and freely. It can't move, because its roots are deep in the ground, and it can't grow upward due to being constantly pruned—usually by relatives or close friends. Since Lowers put a high priority on family, they are more susceptible to being negatively affected or limited by the desires of their tribe.

SPLIT CHAKRA TYPE

Splits are actually quite close to being fully balanced, because they have developed all (or most) of their chakras, in both the upper and lower parts of their energy field, except for one: the solar plexus.

Splits often have an unusually strong desire to love and be loved that causes them to compromise their fiery solar plexus chakra. The third chakra is the home of ego, anger, power, judgment, and selfishness, so it's understandable that Splits, who are very heart-centered, generally want to stay away from it.

Here are some of the beliefs I've heard from Splits that keep them from embracing their solar plexus chakra:

- If I take care of myself first, others will think I'm selfish.
- If I take charge, others will think I'm bossy.
- If I get angry, I'll hurt somebody or get rejected.

- If I'm really myself, nobody will love me.
- If I don't sacrifice myself, I'm not a good person.

Because Split Chakra Types have a heart/solar plexus imbalance, they usually end up as caretakers and people-pleasers who want to be seen as "nice," and avoid confrontation at all costs. This then saps them of their personal power, which makes them even less in touch with what they really want and who they really are. It becomes a negatively reinforced spiral.

For this reason, Splits are often confused, unsure, and unclear about what they want, and find it difficult to make decisions. This leads them into either simultaneously experiencing contradictory feelings like anxiety and depression or into having contrasting experiences back-to-back. For instance, Splits might make a lot of money and then lose it all, or lose a lot of weight, and then gain it all back.

A good metaphor for the Split is a wobbly spinning top. Because they tend to avoid their solar plexus chakra, they don't have the strong center they need to deal with the forces around them. If someone sets them spinning, they tend to be confused, discombobulated, and indecisive. If they can strengthen their solar plexus chakra and own their own

fire power, they will suddenly find that they can direct their own "spin" and also their destiny.

MAIN CHAKRA TYPE HYBRIDS

If your chakras are beautifully balanced, you won't fall into any of the main chakra types, because they were created to assess and remedy common patterns of chakra imbalance.

If you have chakra imbalances that don't seem to fit into these categories, you may be a hybrid of two of these chakra types.

I find that most people fall into a hyphenate category like Lower–Split or Split–Upper. The first part of the hyphenate is the strongest aspect. For instance, an Upper–Split has the qualities of both types, but is more Upper than Split.Lower–Split or Split–Upper. The first part of the hyphenate is the strongest aspect. For instance, an Upper–Split has the qualities of both types, but is more Upper than Split.

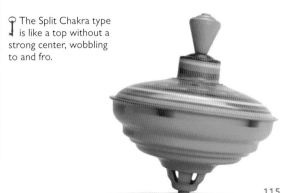

The Split Chakra type is like a top without a strong center, wobbling to and fro.

WHAT CHAKRA TYPE ARE YOU?

UPPER DOMINANT	LOWER DOMINANT
Moves quickly	Moves slowly (or is stuck)
Tends toward anxiety	Tends toward depression
Has more freedom than money	Has more money than freedom
Loves experience most	Loves material things
Loves change/hates routine	Loves the known/hates change
Trusts easily and too much	Trusts slowly and too little
Talks more	Talks less
Lighter/taller/can't gain	Heavier/shorter/easy to gain
Decides quickly	Decides slowly
Fears commitment	Commits strongly
Scattered/accident prone	Solid/safety oriented

TO HEAL	TO HEAL
Grounding and gardening	Enlightenment activities
Drumming and didgeridoo	Prayer, gratitude, meditation
Do pottery and create routines	Movement, celebration
Commitment to repetition	Take risks and change beliefs
Emphasize BODY	Emphasize SPIRIT

SPLIT

Tries not to move

Bounces back and forth (bipolar)

Tends to make money and lose it

Vacillates: experiences and things

Loves/hates routine and change

Trust levels vacillate

Talks only when feels accepted

Weight tends to vacillate

Stays undecided/confused

Has trouble acting on word

Usually more safe than risky

TO HEAL

Motivate and build confidence

Pilates and core yoga

Inner child work and firewalking

Take action (any action!)

Emphasize bridging BODY–SPIRIT

TIME FOR HEALING

Now that you have all the tools you need to properly assess your chakras, you can get a good snapshot of what is going on in your energy field and where you may be habitually shutting down. This is the golden key. Because once you know where you tend to close down, you know where you need to open up to access your innate wholeness.

I recommend trying different methods of assessment. This helps you discover the ones with which you most resonate, and also gives you a way of cross-validating your results. Since most of us can't actually see our chakras, we sometimes doubt our own assessments. When the same chakra comes up as underactive or overactive in many different assessments, it gives you the clarity (or wake-up call) you need to confidently dedicate yourself to healing it.

When you are clear on which chakras need the most attention for systemic balance, you're ready to begin your healing. In chapter three, we're going to explore many different healing options and identify the best methods for each chakra.

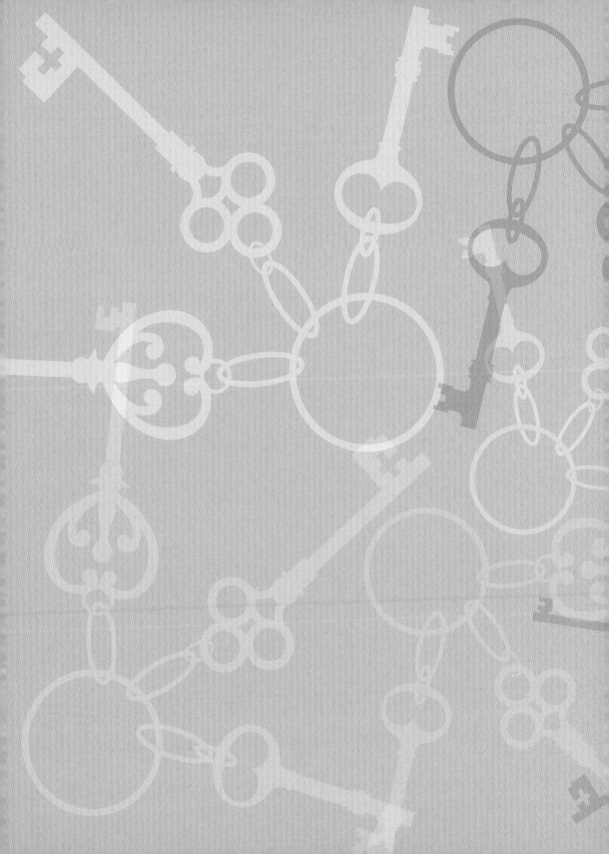

CHAPTER THREE

THE KEY to HEALING YOUR CHAKRAS

- Discover the Most Essential Element for Healing

- Heal Your Chakras with Aromas, Sound, Crystals, and More

- Find Out which Yoga Moves and Poses Open Each Chakra

- Use Your Chakras to Evolve and Live Your Highest Potential

THE MOST ESSENTIAL PART OF HEALING

There are all sorts of effective modalities you can use to boost, balance, and heal your chakras. Some will resonate deeply with you, and others, not as much. Ultimately, it's up to you to choose what works best for you and create your own healing journey. The thing I want to emphasize more than anything else, though, is that none of the methods in this book will balance your chakras without the most essential ingredient: your intention to heal and embody your innate spiritual wholeness.

KEEPING THE RIGHT MINDSET

When it comes to energy healing, your intention and overall mindset is everything. You can engage in all sorts of healing modalities without the right intention and nothing will change.

Conversely, you can simply think about healing your energy field with loving intention, and you'll shift in positive ways.

Every day is a new opportunity to set a powerful intention for healing.

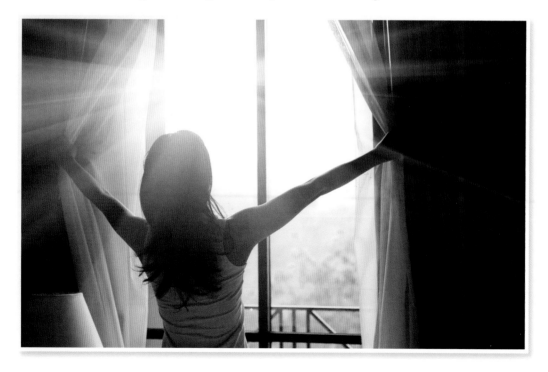

This is due to the fact that intention literally steers energy. It is the driver that tells your energy what to do. And it also motivates you to take the consistent actions you need to make in order for your chakra healings to stick. The goal is not just for you to positively shift the energy of your field, but to create a healthier way of being that becomes your new norm.

Some people promote the idea that energy healing can be instantaneous, and indeed it can. But this kind of instant change often shifts back to its previous state. In order for a positive energetic change to become your new normal, it typically needs reinforcement through repetition.

In other words, our spiritual nature is capable of absolutely anything, but instantaneous changes only last and

permeate our body when we commit to them and repeat them until they turn into our new habits.

THE VALUE OF SHIFTING YOUR PATTERNS

When working with different chakra healing modalities, be aware that you will tend to subconsciously avoid the modalities you need the most. This is because your body likes to do what it has always done. Your temperature, blood pressure, and resting heart beat are constantly trying to find homeostasis. But chakra healing often calls for you to do what you never do, so you can balance out the one-sided nature of your daily habits.

One very popular new-age adage is "Do what you love." While that's certainly good advice some of the time, it's not very wise to heed it all of the time. More of the same will just lead to more of the same. If you really want things to change, you need to change the things you do.

KEYNOTE

The right mindset for chakra healing starts with a clear, unwavering intention to heal. That leads to deep commitment, which turns into focused action, and the ability to magnetize and utilize every opportunity for healing.

DEALING WITH A HEALING CRISIS

Everybody knows that healing is supposed to make you feel better. But the truth is sometimes an effective healing process will at first make you feel worse. This is due to the fact that as we start to shift our old patterns, our body has to move out of its usual homeostasis, which can create unpleasant, withdrawal-type symptoms such as headaches, rashes, breakouts, dizziness, and more.

It's unfortunate that very few healers openly address this issue, because without any understanding of what a healing crisis is, many people interpret their negative symptoms as a sign they're doing something wrong.

Ironically, going into a healing crisis is a sure sign that the healing is actually working! And if people know this, they will stick to their program. On the other hand, if they're not aware that a healing crisis can happen, and they start feeling worse, they may abandon the process right when they're actually starting to create substantial, positive change.

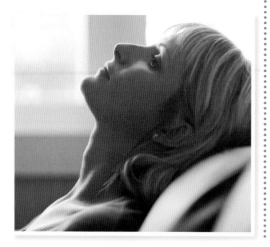

HEALING CRISIS SYMPTOMS

There are three different types of healing crisis symptoms:

- **Ascension Symptoms** (from the energy field moving upward)—headaches and dizziness
- **Grounding Symptoms** (from the energy field moving downward)—extreme tiredness and fatigue.
- **Eliminatory Symptoms** (from getting rid of toxins)—headaches, body achiness, nausea, fatigue, cold and flu symptoms

Regardless of what type of symptoms you're experiencing, the best way to deal with a healing crisis is to follow the five steps in the box on the facing page.

- If you are experiencing ascension symptoms, make an effort to connect more to Mother Earth and do activities like walking in nature, gardening, and drumming. You can also imagine a grounding root extending from your tailbone down to the core of the Earth.

Keep in mind that feeling bad as you begin your healing process may be a good sign.

- If you are experiencing grounding symptoms such as heavy fatigue, try reducing your activity and rest more.
- If you are experiencing elimination symptoms, eat lighter, and drink plenty of really pure water and either turmeric or ginger tea.

FIVE WAYS TO DEAL WITH A HEALING CRISIS

1. **Realize you're having a healing crisis and see it as a sign of growth.** Acknowledge you're going through positive transformation. Symptoms are so much easier to deal with when you see them as a sign of personal progress.

2. **If you're doing a practice or following a program, stick with it.** It's so easy to want to quit a practice when we feel bad. Stay the course during this challenging phase.

3. **Drink more and better water.** Double your normal water intake, and add a little lemon to make it more alkaline.

4. **Breathe more often and more consciously.** It takes real diligence to bring heightened consciousness to breathing, because we are always doing it unconsciously. Consider putting signs up all over the house reminding you to breathe more slowly and deeply.

5. **Carve out more downtime. Rest and sleep more.** If you can create structured time away from work, do that. If not, then take little naps where you can, get more sleep at night, and be gentler with yourself.

In my experience, understanding and accepting that a healing crisis is normal and natural can help you navigate your healing process far more effectively.

Next, we are going to look at the many different ways in which you can heal your chakras.

HEALING THE CHAKRAS WITH AROMATHERAPY

Aromatherapy is one of the easiest and most pleasurable ways to heal your chakras. Odors are around us all the time, and can immediately shift our mood or cause us to recall old memories. This is because aromas affect us on a deep, energetic level. Smell is our most primal sense. Certain scents, like fresh-baked cookies or newly cut grass, can instantaneously take us back to our childhood and others, like the smell of a favorite sweatshirt or a designer cologne, can cause us to suddenly miss someone we love.

Aromas have a way of affecting us on an unconscious, bodily level. They can entice and move us, but beyond that, they can heal us. Smells, just like sounds, have a particular frequency, which means we can use them to target certain chakras or heal our entire energetic field if we set the intention to do so.

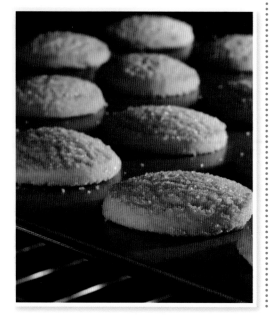

KEYNOTE

Aromatherapy is particularly effective for your root chakra that is associated with your body, memories and sense of smell. So when you want to boost first-chakra qualities like grounding, safety, stability, patience, and endurance, it's one of the best methods you can use, especially if you focus on earthy, woodsy, musky aromas.

For this reason, aromatherapy—the science of using aromas for healing—is a great way to boost and balance your chakras. It's also a great complement to other methods, like visualization, meditation, yoga, massage, crystals, and more.

Nothing smells like home more than your mother's fresh-baked cookies.

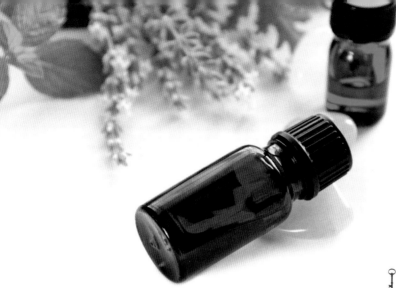

Store your essential oils in darkly tinted bottles to protect them from damaging sunlight.

PRACTICING AROMA AWARENESS

Because the world is filled with different scents, we are all involved in subtle, unofficial forms of aromatherapy every day. We may smell a bouquet of fresh lavender or a cup of steeping chamomile tea and feel more relaxed. Conversely, we may catch the aroma of coffee brewing or smell some strong mint mouthwash, and gain an extra spring in our step.

When you increase your awareness of all the aromas you're exposed to each day and ask yourself if they're beneficial or harmful, you begin activating the power of aromatherapy in your life.

Think about it. How does your partner's cologne make you feel? Are you exposed to the cigarette smoke of a neighbor's apartment? Your coworker's daily tuna sandwich? The smell of gasoline from the station across the way? Do you get out into nature and smell the woodsy scent of trees, moss, and roots? Are you married to a baker who showers you with oven-fresh aromas? In general, do you remember to conjure up the daily smells you love and to avoid the ones that make you cringe?

Since we are exposed to various odors all of our waking hours, becoming aware of the smells that are habitually affecting us, and reinforcing or changing them, can help us to feel happier, healthier, and more balanced.

THE MOST EFFECTIVE ESSENTIAL OILS FOR EACH CHAKRA

The most direct and effective way to tap into the power of aromatherapy is to work with essential oils because each scent activates and balances specific chakras. Some oils heal several or all of the chakras. In this section, I share the most effective oils for each chakra. To avoid repetition, I only associate each oil with one or two of the chakras it affects the most.

ROOT CHAKRA ESSENTIAL OILS

The root chakra is connected to Mother Earth, masculine sexuality, robust systemic health, and grounding. You can heal and balance it best with earthy, musky scents.

- Many of the tree or wood-related oils, like **sandalwood, cedarwood, rosewood,** and **black spruce,** are healing for the root because they bring in strong, grounding energy. Black spruce is also good for relieving muscular aches.
- **Patchouli** heals athlete's foot and also happens to be a powerful aphrodisiac. **Vetiver,** another aphrodisiac, is great for healing the first chakra because it's really safe and non-irritating, and it heals wounds and scars by creating new tissue.

SACRAL CHAKRA ESSENTIAL OILS

Since the sacral chakra is the home of the Divine Feminine and romantic sexuality, sweet, flowery scents and romantic aphrodisiacs are the most therapeutic ones here.

- **Ylang ylang, jasmine, rose,** and **orange blossom** are all aphrodisiacs. Ylang ylang has a densely sweet aroma and is said to reduce any anxiety related to sexual performance. Orange blossom, which is also known as neroli, smells bitter-sweet and has a gentle, sedative effect.
- **Sage, fennel,** and rose all promote good feminine sexual health by stimulating and regulating menstruation. Sage activates the feminine hormone, estrogen, while fennel boosts female libido, and reduces the negative side-effects of menstruation. And rose is such a great tonic for the uterus that it can even delay the onset of menopause.

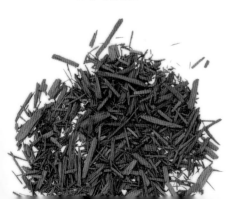

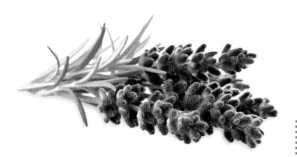

SOLAR PLEXUS CHAKRA ESSENTIAL OILS

The third chakra is about fire, mental clarity, and digestion, so spicy, uplifting, and tummy-soothing scents are the ones to use here.

- **Ginger, black pepper, cardamom, myrrh,** and **peppermint** are all great for healing digestive issues. Ginger is one of the best essential oils for alleviating nausea. Black pepper and myrrh remove gases from the stomach and cardamom is perfect for the fiery third chakra because it literally heats your body up and is good for clearing chest colds.
- **Lemon** and **sage** oil lift both mood and energy and bring mental clarity. They help with digestion and diarrhea, too.
- **Pine** oil increases metabolism and helps you boost your activity levels. It's also great for treating food poisoning.

HEART CHAKRA ESSENTIAL OILS

The heart chakra relates to love and equanimity as well as heart and lung health, immunity, and breathing. Any aromas that strengthen the heart, boost immunity, or facilitate better breathing are great for your fourth chakra.

- **Rosemary** was used by the Ancients as a symbol of love, and it also purifies the air and prevents infections.
- **Thyme** boosts the immune system and strengthens the respiratory system with its antiseptic, antibacterial, and expectorant properties.
- **Ylang ylang** is known to slow down accelerated breathing and heartbeat.
- **Cypress** is considered a respiratory tonic. It tones up the respiratory system and increases efficiency of the lungs.
- **Ginger** and **tea tree** oil are both expectorants. They heal respiratory issues including coughing, asthma, and bronchitis.
- **Eucalyptus** is broadly known for its ability to reduce the symptoms of asthma and other respiratory ailments.

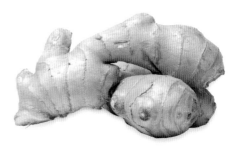

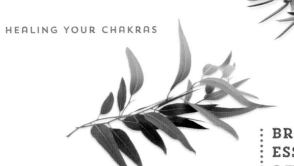

THROAT CHAKRA ESSENTIAL OILS

The fifth chakra relates to your ears, mouth, and throat, as well as purifying your system.

- **Clove oil** has long been used for all sorts of dental care such as treating toothache, sore gums, mouth ulcers, and even cavities. Gargling it with warm water eases throat pain too.
- **Eucalyptus** is often used as a gargle for sore throats as well. And it also helps open the chest and sinuses.
- **German** (or **blue**) **chamomile** has soothing, calming properties and is great for treating ear infections—as is **tea tree** oil.
- **Hyssop** provides numerous benefits, many of which have to do with ridding the body of impurities. It clears out gases and phlegm and has both disinfectant and microbial properties.

BROW CHAKRA ESSENTIAL OILS

The third eye is about good mental balance and eye health, so any oils that relate to your mind's equilibrium or your eyesight are a good fit.

- **Melissa** oil (also known as "sweet oil") comes from the buds and twigs of a Mediterranean plant. It has a soothing, memory boosting, and antidepressant effect.
- **Juniper** oil comes from the purple berries and twigs of the juniper bush. It helps reduce anxiety, insomnia, and mental fatigue.
- **Palmarosa** is a type of grass, but got its name because it smells a lot like rose oil. It fights both depression and anxiety, so it has a balancing, mood-lifting affect.
- **Clary sage** is known for its ability to improve vision and ward against eye issues due to aging. It also has sedative and euphoric effects.
- **Frankincense** has been shown to improve eye health as well.

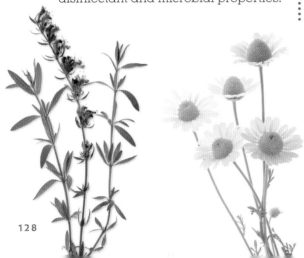

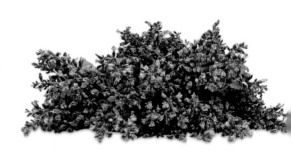

CROWN CHAKRA ESSENTIAL OILS

The highest chakra is about cultivating good mental health and creating a strong connection to the spiritual realm. Some of the essential oils that open and heal the crown are considered holy, and have been used for millennia.

- **Frankincense** has been burned in incense form in churches—from Egyptian to Catholic— throughout history. It has the ability to slow and deepen the breath, which means it is the perfect oil for facilitating meditative states.
- **Helichrysum** has an uplifting effect on mental function and improves energy flow along the meridians of the body.
- **Lavender** is great for any ailment of the nerves or brain. It soothes migraines and reduces anxiety, insomnia, and fainting spells.
- **Rose** is the highest frequency essential oil (according to Bruce Tanio's BT3 Frequency Monitoring System, a sensor he invented to measure the frequency of any substance or object). For this reason, it resonates with the highest chakra.

ESSENTIAL OILS FOR EACH CHAKRA

ROOT CHAKRA
Black spruce
Cedarwood
Patchouli
Rosewood
Sandalwood
Vetiver

HEART CHAKRA
Cypress
Eucalyptus
Ginger
Rosemary
Tea tree
Thyme
Ylang ylang

SACRAL CHAKRA
Fennel
Jasmine
Orange blossom (neroli)
Rose
Sage
Ylang ylang

THROAT CHAKRA
Clove
Eucalyptus
Blue chamomile
Hyssop
Tea tree

SOLAR PLEXUS CHAKRA
Black pepper
Cardamom
Ginger
Lemon
Myrrh
Peppermint
Pine
Sage

BROW CHAKRA
Clary sage
Frankincense
Juniper
Melissa
Palmarosa

CROWN CHAKRA
Frankincense
Helichrysum
Lavender
Rose

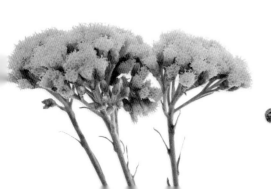
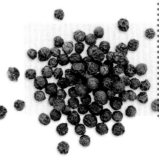

HOW TO USE ESSENTIAL OILS

There are three distinct ways you can enjoy the benefits of essential oils. You can use them topically, that is by applying them to your skin, use them aromatically, or (with properly approved oils only!) you can even ingest them. Whatever method you choose to use, start by purchasing some high-quality therapeutic essential oils. Many of the scented oils that are used for cosmetics, soaps, and other products have a nice smell, but don't carry the healing frequencies of therapeutic oils.

If you're on a budget, make sure to spend enough to get good-quality essential oils, and then save money on the carrier oil you use for diluting it. Whenever possible, use organic carrier oil, and always make sure that it's not rancid before adding in the more expensive essential oil.

Some of the most popular carrier oils are jojoba, grapeseed, or coconut oil. Extra virgin, cold-pressed olive oil is also an affordable option.

Peppermint essential oil can soothe an upset stomach and boost your solar plexus chakra.

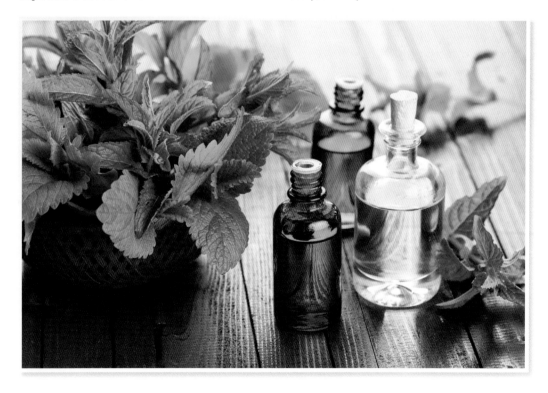

Always store your essential oils in a cool, dry place away from light, and make sure they're covered securely after use. Never store them in a plastic container, as the oils can break down some of the toxic ingredients in the plastic.

If you use coconut oil as a carrier, use the fractionated kind if you want it to stay liquid.

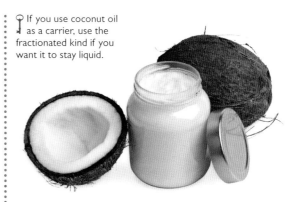

USING ESSENTIAL OILS TOPICALLY

One easy way to use essential oils is to dilute them and put them on your skin. This works well for chakra healing, since you can put the oil related to a particular chakra right where that chakra is located.

The recipe for diluting varies among aromatherapy practitioners. A common amount of dilution is 5–10 drops of essential oil to an ounce of carrier oil, but some people who like to work with superpotent essential oils will use up to a 50:50 mix.

To determine the right dilution for you, do a skin test. Simply put a small amount of diluted oil on the area of your elbow crease and see if you get any reaction (like redness or rash). If there is none, you can then use that essential oil for healing.

Keep in mind that the less you dilute an essential oil, the more likely it is to create a skin reaction. Also, everybody has a different level of skin sensitivity. So if you change the strength of an oil mixture or you use a diluted essential oil on a different person, do a new skin test.

Another topical way you can enjoy essential oils is by putting them in your bath. Generally, it's not good to put them directly in your bath, since oil pockets can float in the water without ever being diluted and can irritate the skin.

A better way to use essential oils in the bath is to make your own bath salts (see page 132). It's easy, and the salts you use with the oils are very healing as well.

Some of the most popular essential oils for making bath salts are:
- **Energizing:** Spearmint and rosemary
- **Relaxing:** Lavender and frankincense
- **Mood Lifting:** Lemon and tangerine
- **Reducing Aches:** Eucalyptus

HOW TO MAKE YOUR OWN ESSENTIAL OIL BATH SALTS

GATHER THESE INGREDIENTS

- 1 cup (270 g) of Epsom or Himalayan salts, or sea salt (or a mix)
- 20 drops of essential oils (one type or a blend)
- 1 teaspoon of jojoba, grapeseed, or coconut oil

1. Mix the essential oil(s) with the carrier oil(s). Next, add the salt and stir well.

2. When done, put it all into an airtight glass container for when you're ready to use it. If you want to create a larger batch, simply multiply the recipe.

NOTE: If you would like to add a little fizz to your bath, stir in 2 teaspoons of baking soda after the salt has absorbed all of the oil.

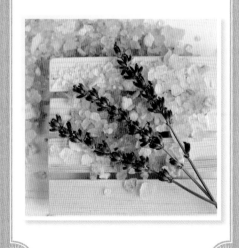

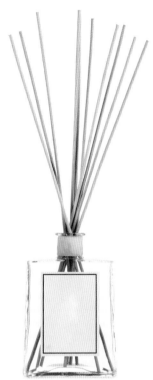

Reed diffusers are a cheap and simple way to fill a room with essential oil aromas.

USING ESSENTIAL OILS AROMATICALLY

Another great way to benefit from essential oils is to smell them. You can simply take a whiff of any oil right from the container, or you can put a small amount on your palms, rub them together, and lightly cup your hands around your nose for a really potent hit. If you are skin sensitive, be sure to skin test an oil before putting it on your palms.

You can also use a diffuser to spread the scent and benefits of your essential oils throughout a room. There are several different kinds: cool mist, steam-based, reed, and even some that sit on the top of a lamp where the heat of the lightbulb diffuses the oil.

INGESTING ESSENTIAL OILS

There is much debate around whether essential oils can be ingested safely. They are totally natural, but they are also extremely concentrated and potent. If you choose to consume them, you should stick to the oils that relate to stomach issues and only in very small quantities when properly diluted.

Because water and oil do not mix, you can dilute them by mixing 1 drop of essential oil into 1 teaspoon of honey, and then adding that mixture to a cup of warm water.

The safest way of all to ingest essential oils is to buy a blend made specifically for that purpose. One of the world's biggest suppliers of essential oils, Young Living, creates a whole line of essential oils that are meant to be ingested. All of their edible oils have a name that ends with "Vitality." For instance, they offer both a Peppermint essential oil (which is not edible), and a Peppermint Vitality that you can ingest.

Lavender oil is edible when properly diluted and used in very small quantities.

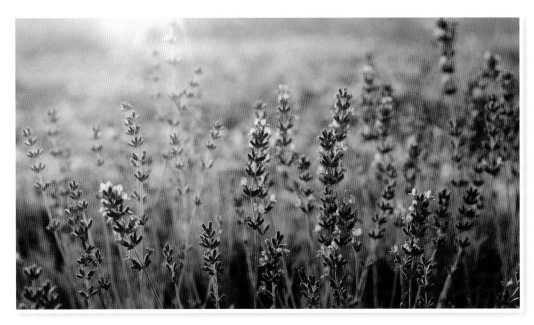

HEALING THE CHAKRAS WITH SOUND

Everyone intuitively knows that sound can be healing or disruptive. From the soothing lap of waves on a shore or a cat's gentle purring to the disturbing shriek of a piercing scream or fingernails scraping on a chalkboard, sound can elicit a whole spectrum of responses. We might recoil from an angry reprimand, swoon over an exquisite aria, get motivated by a marching band, or sleep more sweetly while serenaded by a chorus of crickets. Sound affects us deeply and instantaneously, because it literally changes our vibration. And, since vibration is the essence of all creation, sound healing goes straight to the underlying cause of illness and disease.

Many different world religions embrace the idea that the word is associated with God and the power of creation. Hindu scripture claims that the whole word is in the syllable "om" and the Christian bible says that first there was the Word, and out of it, everything else was created. This is because sound has an underlying structure that compels consciousness to take form.

PATTERNS OF SACRED GEOMETRY

It seems that the power of vibration is one of the rare areas where religion and science actually agree. In the 1800s, German scientist Ernst Chladni carried out experiments where he played a violin bow along the edge of a steel plate full of sand, and beautiful mandala-like patterns formed in the sand. Each time Chladni played a different frequency, he got a different design.

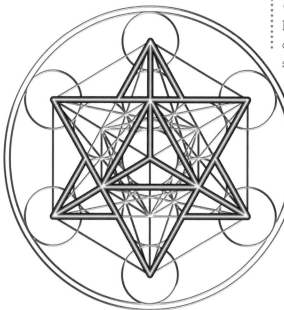

Sacred geometry recognizes sacred universal patterns in everything in our reality.

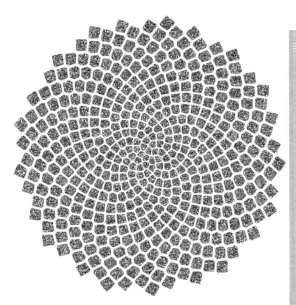

Vibrating sound waves can produce extraordinary symmetrical patterns—a phenomenon known as cymatics.

Since that time, the phenomenon that came to be known as cymatics has been replicated in many other experiments. It has become very clear that when sound waves are projected into various physical media, such as powder, water, oils, and more, beautiful patterns of sacred geometry arise.

Sound literally has a formative effect on matter, and it's not a chaotic or random effect. The results are always patterned and predictable. Lower vibrations cause a different pattern than higher sounds and repeating the exact same vibration will create an identical pattern.

SIMPLE SOUND PATTERN EXERCISE

You can create your own cymatics using just a drum and a speaker and following these simple steps.

YOU WILL NEED
- An open-bottom drum
- A speaker
- A music source
- Poppy seeds, salt, or flour

1. Place the drum over a speaker so that the sound can move up into the drum.

2. Sprinkle a layer of poppy seeds, salt, or flour on the top of the drum.

3. Play frequencies through the speaker with an electric keyboard or tone generator (with the goal of creating a waveform signal at a specific pitch). If you don't have these, try using digital recordings of single pitches.

4. Play different pitches and take pictures of the different patterns formed in your seeds, salt, or flour.

EVERYDAY SOUND HEALING

Sound healing works via your throat chakra and the fifth layer of your aura, the Etheric Template. This is the place in your energy field where all manifestation begins and it's the reason that all sounds, including language, are powerful tools for creating positive, physical change.

The concept of sound healing applies to an extremely wide range. It can be as formal as a healer playing specific frequencies on a sacred instrument like a harp, crystal bowl, or didgeridoo, or as informal as someone singing along to a recording of their favorite song.

For this reason, it's an intuitive process, and one of the simplest, most important questions you can ask yourself regarding sound healing is: Does this sound or music make me feel better? Does it bring me into a more balanced, happier, or more loving state?

Anything that puts you into the sweet spot of your heart chakra creates more balance in your chakra system, because your heart is the equalizing, center chakra of your energy field.

So, for overall, general healing, the key is to find music or sounds that bring you into your heart and make you happier. Similarly, you want to limit your exposure to sounds that make you feel stressed, agitated, depressed, or cause you to experience any other negative state.

Whether or not you choose to engage in formal sound-healing sessions, it will definitely benefit you to pay more attention to the sounds in your life, and see whether yours are healing and balancing, or disruptive and damaging.

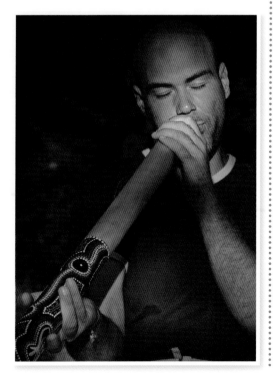

The didgeridoo is a powerful root chakra instrument of Aboriginal origin.

EXERCISE TO INCREASE YOUR SOUND AWARENESS

1. Wherever you are, read these steps, then close your eyes and listen closely.

2. What do you hear? Notice and name the different sounds.

3. How do they make you feel? Calm? Happy? Agitated? Or… ?

4. Are they loud and close or quiet and distant?

5. Do any of the sounds bring up memories? If so, what are they?

6. Ask your intuition: Is this a healing sound environment, or not?

7. If it is not a healing environment, ask yourself if you can add or remove some sounds (for example, hanging chimes outside your kitchen window or calming a barking dog).

8. Or, if you are in a temporary environment, give yourself conscious permission to leave and find a better option.

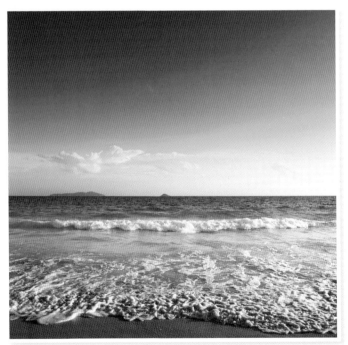

CHAKRA HEALING NOTES AND MANTRAS

Because sound is vibratory and organized in a way that is similar to the chakras, there are many ways it can be used for chakra healing. At its most basic, each chakra corresponds to a note on the musical scale, with base note "C" corresponding to the root chakra. Working up through the rest of the chakras, "D" is associated with the sacral chakra, "E" with the solar plexus chakra, and so on up the scale.

The fact that each chakra corresponds to a note means that singing a song like "Do Re Mi" from the musical *The Sound of Music* can literally balance your chakras. No wonder so many people adore the movie!

Still, the notes we are talking about for chakra healing are not the notes of your average piano (which uses a C note that vibrates at 261 Hz), but those of an ancient scale known as the Solfeggio Frequencies that start with a C note at 256 Hz, a frequency many claim is the resonance of Earth itself. Solfeggio frequencies comprise six pure tonal notes and are used in Gregorian Chant and other forms of sacred music.

HEALING NOTES

The best way to use musical notes for chakra healing is to buy a set of tuning forks or crystal bowls specifically designed to cover all seven chakras. When you want to heal a particular chakra, you can place the appropriate bowl or tuning fork right on that chakra and strike it to create curative sound. Or, if you are doing a sound healing for a group, you can simply play the instrument for everyone.

Each healing bowl or tuning fork not only plays a particular note, it also resonates at a particular Solfeggio

The original Solfeggio scale was devised by an 11th-century monk, Guido d'Arezzo, to make the task of learning songs and chants easier.

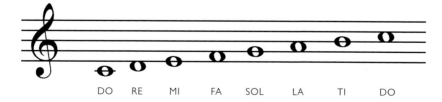

DO   RE   MI   FA   SOL   LA   TI   DO

frequency that corresponds to its note. The Solfeggio frequencies are the most popular among chakra healers, but there are other systems you can use.

The best rule of thumb with sound healing is to consult your intuition. Feel into how each vibration, sound, or instrument resonates for you. When I went to buy a Tibetan singing bowl, I was intuitively drawn to one that I later discovered has a heart frequency. When I play it, I feel calmer and more centered.

HEALING MANTRAS

The Sanskrit word "mantra" is comprised of "man," meaning "mind," and "tra," which translates as "protect or defend." Mantras are tools that help us protect our mind from scattered or negative thought patterns.

Traditionally, mantras are sacred Sanskrit words that are repeated for healing purposes. In reality, though, any word or sound that carries a positive resonance and is sustainably repeated can have the same powerful, therapeutic effect.

KEYNOTE

Crystal bowls can be very expensive, so if you're on a limited budget, consider using Tibetan bowls that are made from a mix of copper and tin and cost far less.

It's important to realize that a mantra does not get its power from intellectual recognition of a word. You do not need to know the literal meaning of a word for it to work as a mantra. Its power comes from its vibration. In fact, not knowing the definition of a mantra can prove helpful, because it doesn't stir up any thoughts or mind chatter.

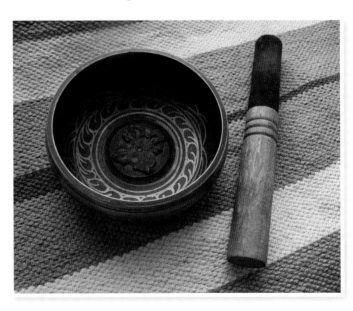

Tibetan singing bowls, which have been used by monks for centuries, often have sacred engravings.

OM: THE UNIVERSAL MANTRA

There are mantras for health, wealth, love, luck, and even ones for curing snake bites. Perhaps the most well-known mantra of all time is "om." Many claim it is the primordial sound that represents absolutely everything from Alpha to Omega. Some say that if you are sensitive enough, you can hear a Universal Om in the background of all existence. In any case, om is a powerful, basic mantra you can use when you want to move your mind away from a mish-mash of scattered thoughts and focus on the Divine.

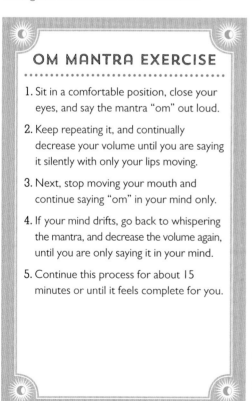

OM MANTRA EXERCISE

1. Sit in a comfortable position, close your eyes, and say the mantra "om" out loud.

2. Keep repeating it, and continually decrease your volume until you are saying it silently with only your lips moving.

3. Next, stop moving your mouth and continue saying "om" in your mind only.

4. If your mind drifts, go back to whispering the mantra, and decrease the volume again, until you are only saying it in your mind.

5. Continue this process for about 15 minutes or until it feels complete for you.

SEED SOUNDS AND NAMES

One simple, vocal way to heal your chakras with sound is to repeatedly chant the seed sound related to each one (see the chart on the facing page). A seed sound is the basic mantra that represents the essence of a thing.

You can focus on one seed sound to boost a specific chakra, or you can say (or sing) all of them sequentially to balance your whole energy field. If you want to boost your liberating current, say them from the bottom up, and if you want to create more manifesting energy, repeat them from the top down.

USING SANSKRIT NAMES

Another related, very powerful way to tap into the energy of a particular chakra is to say its Sanskrit name. Psychics often use someone's name to tap into their energy, because a name holds the essence of the thing it represents. You can boost and balance a chakra by repeatedly chanting or saying its name with devotion. I repeat the name of each chakra in every song on my healing album, *Chakra Love*. On the next page I have provided the chakra Sanskrit names with a guide on how to pronounce them.

CHAKRA SOUND CORRESPONDENCES

Chakra Sound	Note	Seed	Frequency	Music Type	Nature Sound
Root	C	Lam	256 Hz	Tribal	Landslide/quake
Sacral	D	Vam	288 Hz	Jazz	Ocean
Solar Plexus	E	Ram	320 Hz	Rock	Fire/volcano
Heart	F	Yam	341.3 Hz	Easy listening	Wind
Throat	G	Ham	384 Hz	Opera	Thunder
Brow	A	Om	426.7 Hz	Choral	Birds
Crown	B	Silence	480 Hz	Classical	Universal Om

SANSKRIT CHAKRA NAMES
- **Root Chakra:** Muladhara (moo-luh-dar-uh)
- **Sacral Chakra:** Svaddisthana (svah-dee-stah-nuh)
- **Solar Plexus:** Manipura (mah-nee-pure-uh)
- **Heart Chakra:** Anahata (ahn-uh-ha-tuh)
- **Throat Chakra:** Visuddha (vis-shoo-duh)
- **Brow Chakra:** Ajna (ahj-nuh)
- **Crown Chakra:** Sahasrara (sah-haz-rah-rah)

DEITY MANTRAS
Finally, one last way you can use mantras to heal your chakras is to repeat ones that are related to the Hindu gods or goddesses associated with each chakra. If you resonate with a particular spiritual entity or archetype, doing this kind of mantra can bring in a powerful element of devotion that increases the mantra's effect.

There are several different spiritual deities associated with each chakra and there are many different mantras for each deity, so the chart shown here is in no way definitive. It's just a good place to start. You can search the internet for more mantras or even create some of your own. You can use one of these two basic salutatory mantras and simply insert the name of a deity you want to honor:

Om Namah [deity] ya Swaha.

Om Shree [deity], Jaya [deity].

Om is the ultimate sound of everything. Shree (also "shri") is a word you put before someone's name as a sign of respect, as is namah, which means "to bow to." Jaya means "victory," which is why it works best for the deities of the masculine chakras, and swaha is a word that you put at the end of a mantra to show faith and completion. It is akin to "and so it is."

HEALING DEITIES

Lakshmi is the beautiful Goddess of abundance and **Rati** is the enchanting Goddess of sexuality, love, and partnership.

Lord Rama is one of the incarnations of the Hindu god Vishnu. He's a strong choice for the solar plexus chakra, because his name includes the seed sound for the core's energy center. Another option for the third chakra is to honor **Surya**, the god of the sun.

Hanuman is the loving and humble monkey-god that loyally served Lord Rama. He is known for his unparalleled heart.

Vaka (or Vac) is the secret goddess of the voice and **Mahadevi** stands for the "Great Mother," and includes all of the

CHAKRA DEITY MANTRAS

Chakra	God/Goddess	Mantra
Root	Lakshmi	Om Shreem Maha Laksmiyay Swaha
Sacral	Rati	Om Shree Maha Ratiyay Swaha
Solar Plexus	Rama	Om Shree Rama, Jaya Rama
Heart	Hanuman	Om Namah Hanumante Swaha
Throat	Vac/Vaka	Om Shree Vaka, Jaya Vaka
Brow	Mahadevi	Om Shreem Mahadeviyay Swaha
Crown	Shiva	Om Namah Shivaya

wisest Hindu goddesses. Lord **Shiva** is one of the greatest known and revered Hindu gods.

THE POWER OF SILENCE AND RESONANCE

One of the most essential tools of sound healing is silence. Every sound has a vibration and it is this subtle movement, rather than the sound itself, that affects the etheric realm and creates healing.

As you can imagine, in our noisy world, the vibration of silence is one of the most calming and healing of all. This is probably why just 15–20 minutes of silent meditation a day can have profound positive effects on your mind, body, and spirit.

When consciously engaging in sound healing, it's important to keep in mind that there are many sounds we cannot hear that, nevertheless, have a positive or negative effect on our being. We are constantly resonating and entraining with others without any communication or audible sound at all.

All of us have experienced a time when our mood has been lifted or brought down by a friend or partner. And we have created the same effect for others too.

If a group of women live together for a while, they will resonate so perfectly that they'll begin to menstruate in sync.

If you introduce a new woman with an irregular menstrual cycle into the household, after a few cycles, it's quite likely she'll be menstruating right along with the rest. That's how powerful vibrational entrainment can be.

In the purest sense, it's a form of sound healing, because we all continually send out a sort of sonar that is our personal frequency. And we are constantly taking in and adjusting to the personal resonance of others. In any group setting, everyone will eventually entrain with the person who emits the strongest vibration.

Sound healing is a magical realm, a world in which different types of structured vibration like words or music can be used to create more beauty and well-being. Invoke sounds that resonate at the frequencies of your chakras and, over time, you'll create a happier, healthier and more harmonious life.

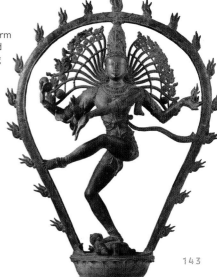

Naraja is a well-known form of the Hindu god Shiva performing the eternal cosmic dance.

HEALING THE CHAKRAS WITH HATHA YOGA

Since yogis were the first ones to describe the chakras thousands of years ago, it shouldn't come as a surprise that Hatha yoga—the practice of doing physical poses—is one of the best ways to boost and balance your chakras. Because our society is so sedentary, most adults need to stretch more. And this causes many people to erroneously believe that the physical practice of yoga is solely about stretching and being flexible. In fact, Hatha yoga is designed to develop both the masculine and feminine aspects of your body. It's true that yoga entails stretching, but it also emphasizes the opposite—making your body stronger and more stable.

Hatha yoga is designed to open and cultivate all of your chakras from the stability of your root to the freedom of your crown, and every state in between. Since our chakras reside in specific areas of our body, we can use different poses to strengthen and open the different parts of our anatomy that relate to each chakra, such as legs for the root chakra, hips for the sacral chakra, core for the solar plexus chakra, and so on.

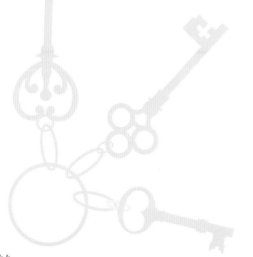

THE YOGIC PRINCIPLES OF ALIGNMENT

It's important to realize that every pose, when done with proper alignment, involves and activates all of your chakras. For this reason, it's preferable to put more focus on the yogic movements of your practice—the Principles of Alignment—than the yoga poses themselves. Because while there are many different poses that are anatomically related to each chakra, energetically, there is only one Principle of Alignment that directly activates each energy center.

When you learn how to perform the specific Principle of Alignment that activates each chakra (described on pages 154–157), you can directly influence any individual chakra in any given pose. This can be very handy when one energy center, in particular, is outof balance.

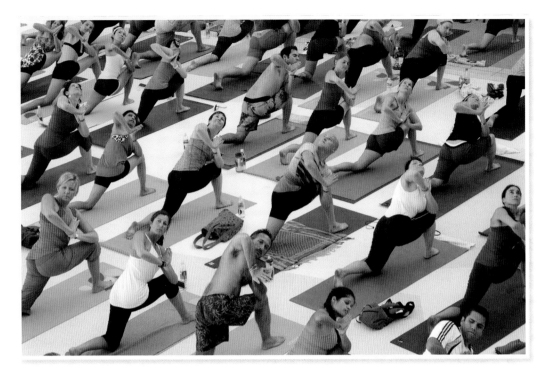

For example, when I had a chronically underactive root chakra, I did a wide variety of yoga poses every day. But with each one, I focused mostly on muscular contraction, the alignment principle related to the root chakra. I made it my main priority in every pose, and gradually my yoga practice, finances, and life in general became stronger and more stable.

Ideally, once you've learned all the Principles of Alignment, you'll do all seven of them in every pose. This will take your practice to a whole new level where you'll experience more energy and flow. The key thing to understand is that the way you do a yoga pose is far

As yoga grows in popularity, so do the big festivals like Wanderlust, shown here.

more important than the specific pose you chose to do. Yoga positions are only the outer shapes you create, while the Principles of Alignment are the physical mechanics that enable you to go deeper than mere anatomy, and tap directly into the energy of each chakra.

First, let's look at a few yoga poses for each chakra. I'm going to give you the most essential, basic poses, but there are still many more you can do. For a comprehensive guide, check out Anodea Judith's *Chakra Yoga*.

ROOT CHAKRA POSES

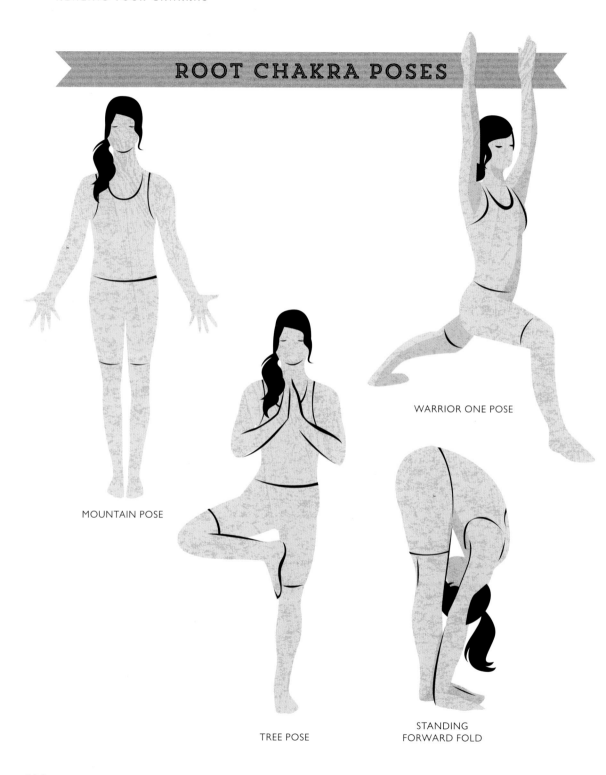

MOUNTAIN POSE

TREE POSE

WARRIOR ONE POSE

STANDING
FORWARD FOLD

SACRAL CHAKRA POSES

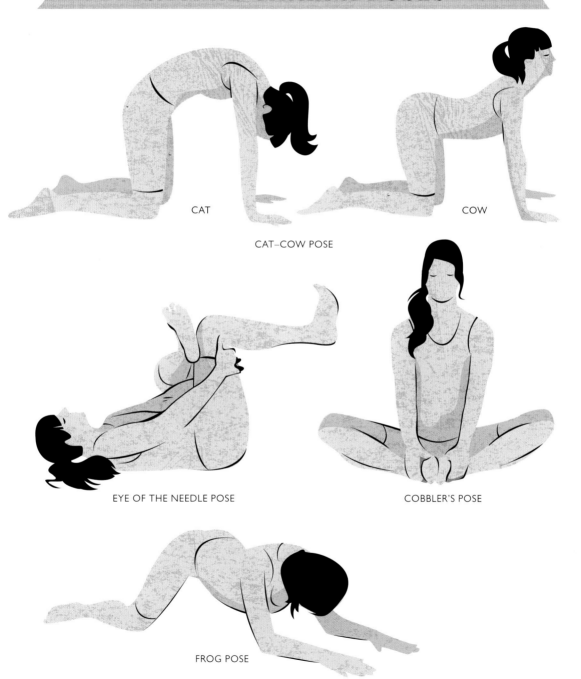

CAT

COW

CAT–COW POSE

EYE OF THE NEEDLE POSE

COBBLER'S POSE

FROG POSE

SOLAR PLEXUS CHAKRA POSES

BALANCING CAT

BOAT POSE
(BENT KNEE
VARIATION)

FOREARM PLANK

UPWARD FACING TABLE POSE

HEART CHAKRA POSES

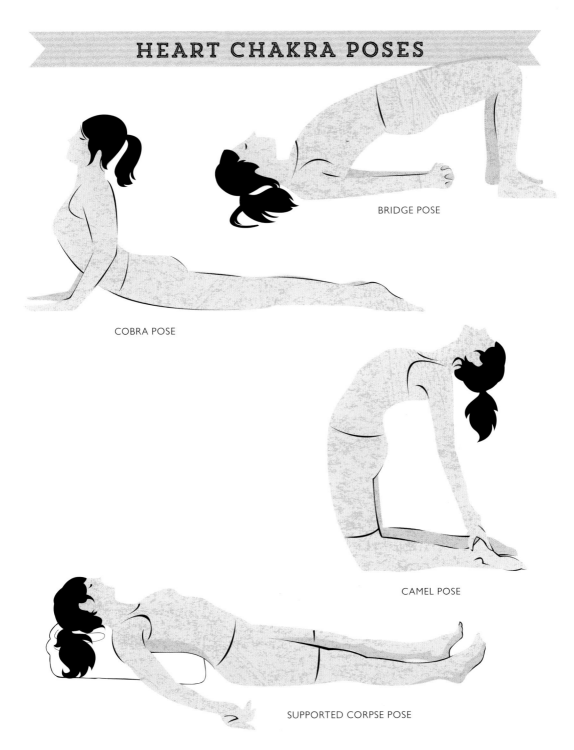

BRIDGE POSE

COBRA POSE

CAMEL POSE

SUPPORTED CORPSE POSE

THROAT CHAKRA POSES

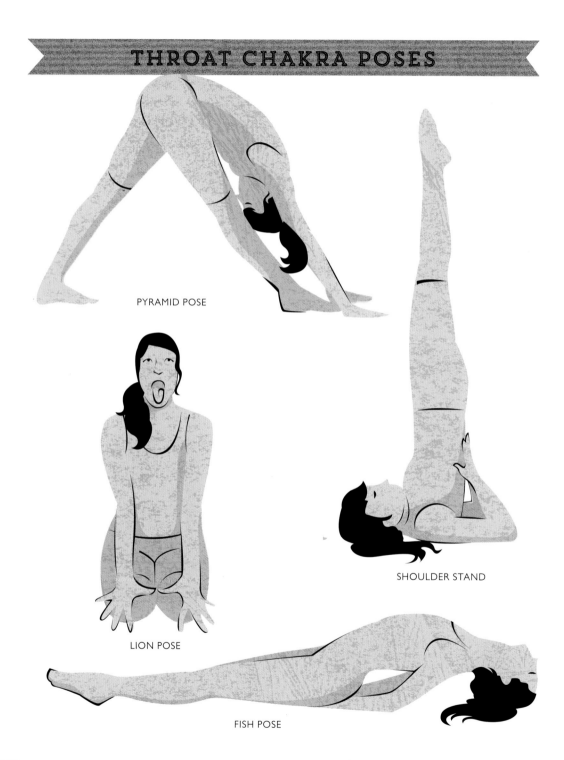

PYRAMID POSE

LION POSE

SHOULDER STAND

FISH POSE

BROW CHAKRA POSES

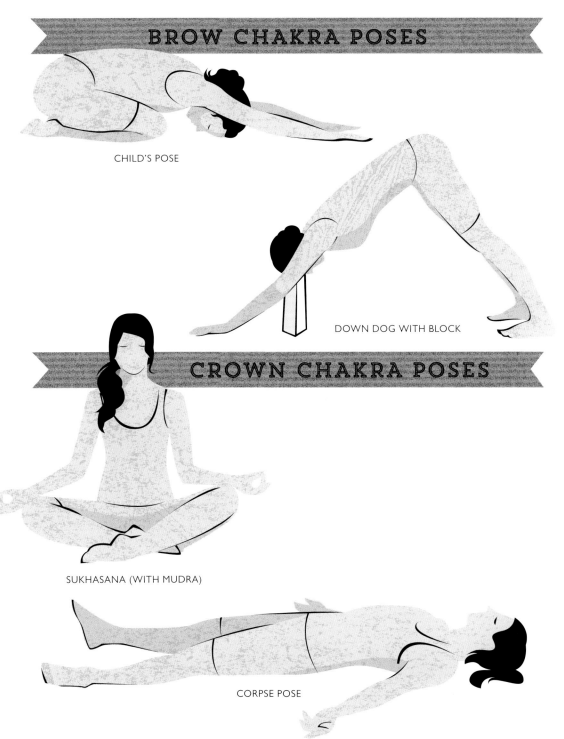

CHILD'S POSE

DOWN DOG WITH BLOCK

CROWN CHAKRA POSES

SUKHASANA (WITH MUDRA)

CORPSE POSE

THE YOGIC PRINCIPLES OF ALIGNMENT

The Yogic Principles of Alignment allow you to access and align all of your chakras in every pose. You want to perform all the principles in every pose. Also, always finish every sequence in Corpse Pose. This allows you to relax and surrender, and gives your body the opportunity to fully integrate your practice.

CHAKRA HEALING THROUGH YOGA

There are two basic, effective ways you can approach chakra healing through yoga:

1. Focus on healing a particular chakra that you know is out of balance and do a series of poses that positively affect it.

2. Focus on balancing your entire energy field and do a sequence that includes one or two poses for each chakra.

Try this sample yoga sequence (right) that moves through all the chakras, created out of the poses shown on pages 146–151. Or get creative and make your own!

SAMPLE YOGA SEQUENCE

- Mountain Pose (*Root and Crown—the best starting pose*)
- Standing Forward Fold (*Root Chakra*)
- Cat–Cow (*Sacral Chakra*)
- Balancing Cat (*Solar Plexus Chakra*)
- Bridge Pose (*Heart Chakra*)
- Shoulder Stand (*Throat Chakra*)
- Child's Pose (*Brow Chakra*)
- Corpse Pose (*Crown Chakra—the best finishing pose*)

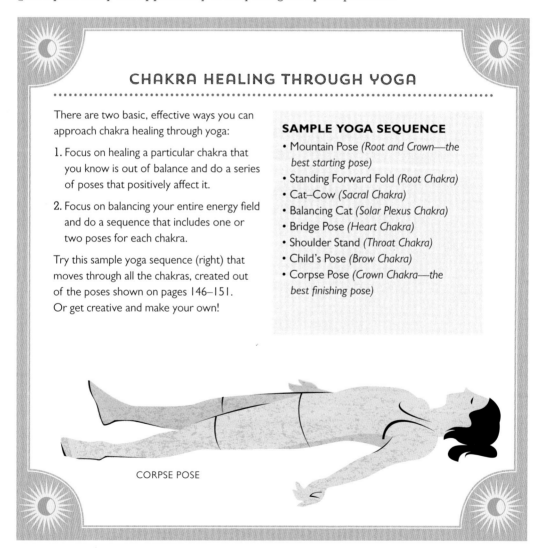

CORPSE POSE

HOW TO BALANCE THE CHAKRAS IN MOUNTAIN POSE

I'm going to show you how to apply the Yogic Principles of Alignment to Mountain Pose, which should give you a good feel for how to apply the principles to most of the basic poses.

Sometimes, I will ask you to make an "isometric" movement. To do this, simply engage your muscles and create physical force as if you're going to move, but do so without actually moving. This tenses the muscles and creates physical and energetic stability.

In the classic version of Mountain Pose, the legs are usually together, but you might want to try a variation with the legs hip-distance apart. This allows you to feel the muscular contraction between your legs, and, also, it creates better alignment with your natural anatomy.

As you can see from the photograph (right), Mountain Pose is a position that we're all in a lot of the time. This means you're actually doing "yoga" every time you're standing! If you bring the Yogic Principles of Alignment into your daily movements and posture, your yoga practice will extend well beyond the limited time you can spend on your mat.

To get into the basic shape of Mountain Pose, simply stand fully upright with your feet together or hip-distance apart and your crown lined up over your groin. With your arms at your sides, lift your chest and rotate your inner arms outward so that your biceps and palms face forward as much as possible.

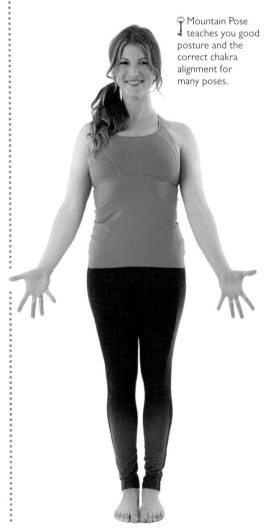

Mountain Pose teaches you good posture and the correct chakra alignment for many poses.

ALIGNMENT PRINCIPLE 1
OPEN TO GRACE (CROWN CHAKRA)

In order to make sure that your yoga practice is energetically based, we need to start with the Yogic Principle of Alignment for the crown chakra: Open to Grace.

Standing in Mountain Pose, simply relax and soften, notice the movement of your breath, and invite Universal energy to fill you up. If you feel like it, you can even imagine your crown opening like a sunroof and allowing light energy to pour in. Once you feel open, soft, and filled with Divine energy, you are ready to build a strong, earthy foundation.

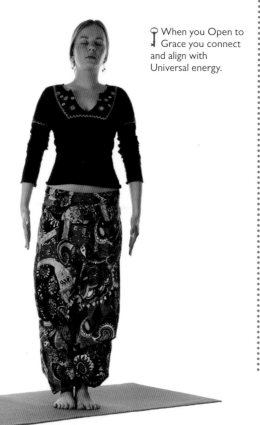

When you Open to Grace you connect and align with Universal energy.

ALIGNMENT PRINCIPLE 2
MUSCULAR CONTRACTION (ROOT CHAKRA)

To have a strong root chakra, you need to create physical stability. Standing in Mountain Pose, lift your toes off the floor, spread them wide, and place them back down to create a solid foundation.

Now, you're ready to engage in Muscular Contraction. There are three different ways you can do it. Practice each one individually, until you can do them all simultaneously:

1. Isometrically draw your legs together toward the midline (without physically moving them). As you do this, you should feel a lift in the floor of your pelvis: this is called "mulabandha" (root lock). If you are familiar with Kegel exercises, root lock is basically the same thing—the squeezing and lifting of the perineum.

2. From your extremities (feet and hands), draw inward isometrically toward the center. In Mountain Pose, keep your arms in the same position but energetically draw inward until you feel your shoulder blades moving toward each other on your back.

3. Isometrically draw all your muscles closer to the bone like an Ace elastic bandage. This one is subtler than the others, so it may be hard to feel. Start by imagining your muscles hugging into your bones tightly and, over time, you'll feel your muscles actually contract more and more.

Always make sure you're Open to Grace before you do Muscular Contraction. If you do the first two Yogic Principles of Alignment in the correct order, your body contracts around the Divine energy and gives it beautiful form. But if you do them in the reverse order, your body contracts prematurely and actually blocks Universal energy from entering.

Also, keep in mind that these Yogic Principles of Alignment are sequential and progressive, so as you apply each one, you continue to activate all the ones that came before it.

ALIGNMENT PRINCIPLE 3
INNER SPIRAL (SACRAL CHAKRA)

♀ Inner Spiral opens your hips in a beautiful, natural way. It's the perfect antidote to our culture's chronic chair sitting. To do it in Mountain Pose, simply keep your legs strong and sturdy, and push the top of your inner thighs back and apart. This will cause your rear end to protrude and the top of your pelvis to tilt forward, creating more curve in your lower back.

ALIGNMENT PRINCIPLE 4
OUTER SPIRAL
(SOLAR PLEXUS CHAKRA)

♂ Just as their names imply, doing Inner Spiral naturally leads to doing Outer Spiral. They are a feminine–masculine pair. Inner Spiral opens the hips and causes the femur bones to go deeper into the hip sockets, and Outer Spiral locks them into this more integrated position.

To do Outer Spiral, make sure to continue to activate Inner Spiral, and then simply scoop your tailbone (move it down and forward), causing your thighs to rotate outwardly as they move forward and apart.

If you are confused by the term "scooping your tailbone," just think of it as the hip thrust that a man does when making love. Only in this case, it's done standing up, and you keep doing the feminine action of pushing your thighs back and apart at the same time.

Done correctly, scooping your tailbone will cause your abdominal muscles to contract inward toward your spine, creating the second yogic lock, "uddiyana bandha" (core lock). You will instantaneously feel more abdominal engagement and physical integrity.

ALIGNMENT PRINCIPLE 5
MUSCULAR EXPANSION (HEART CHAKRA)

From this place of feeling firmly grounded in your legs, open in your hips, and powerfully contracted in your core, you're ready to add the energy of an expanded heart.

The Principle of Alignment here is the opposite of the root chakra's Muscular Contraction. Instead of drawing inward, you expand your energy outward.

From your waist, lift your torso upward so your chest widens and opens. Bend your elbows slightly and externally

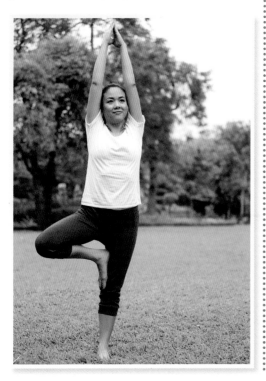

rotate your arms so they face fully forward and then relax your shoulder blades down your back, away from your ears.

Finally, spread your arms and send your energy outward like rays of sunshine from the center of your being.

ALIGNMENT PRINCIPLE 6
THROAT LOCK (THROAT CHAKRA)

After opening your heart, you should be standing tall with a wide, open chest. Drop your chin slightly and contract into your thyroid to create the yogic throat lock (jalandhara bandha). This movement stimulates your thyroid gland that regulates much of your body's hormonal production.

ALIGNMENT PRINCIPLE 7
PALETTE BACK (BROW CHAKRA)

Creating the throat lock tends to pull the head forward, so now you need to get the neck back into alignment. Without losing the contraction of jalandhara bandha, lift your chin slightly and draw the sides of your neck back until your brow chakra aligns over your spine and the rest of your chakras.

Tree Pose is a variation of Mountain Pose that allows you to open your hips and heart.

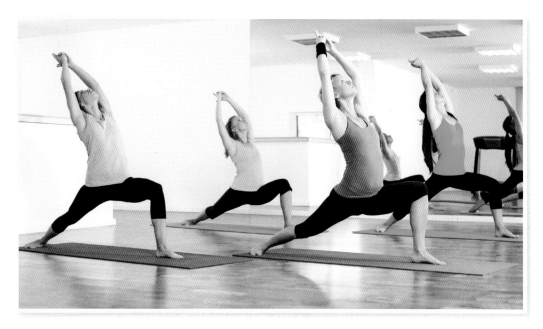

TAKING YOGA BEYOND THE POSES

The physical poses are really only a small part of a much larger yoga discipline that includes breathing, concentrating, and meditating, as well as practicing personal and social ethics. Still, I like to focus on the poses, because they physically shift your body in ways that can keep your chakras balanced for long periods of time.

Many chakra healing methods shift your energy, but don't change your body. If your energy shifts and your body doesn't, then over time, your body will draw your energy back into its old patterns. For instance, if your posture is hunched over, it will be hard for you to keep your heart and solar plexus

Warrior One Pose creates a sense of being simultaneously strong, grounded, and open.

chakras open and strong. If you wear the right stones and aromas and say the right mantras, your heart and core energy can open temporarily. But without the proper posture or movements to physically support and reinforce the new state of your chakras, your body will compel your old energy patterns to return.

If you do yoga regularly, your chakras will move into a pattern of habitual alignment, giving you great posture, too! It takes a big commitment to do yoga consistently, but it's worth it, because it's the one practice that can ensure that your healthier chakra patterns become the new norm for your body.

HEALING THE CHAKRAS WITH CRYSTALS AND GEMSTONES

Laying gemstones on the body for healing purposes has been successfully practiced across numerous cultures for thousands of years. But how can seemingly inert rocks benefit the body? The answer lies in the piezoelectric effect.

To avoid too much technical jargon, you can best understand this scientific phenomenon by considering a quartz watch. When slightly bent, a small piece of quartz puts out a constant voltage that keeps a watch running with phenomenal accuracy. Crystals and gemstones do the same for us. They put out a small charge that interacts with our biomagnetic field and creates more harmony and balance.

HOW TO CHOOSE THE RIGHT STONES FOR YOU

Every stone has a unique vibration, just as every person does. For this reason, the particular stones needed for balancing the chakras will vary somewhat from person to person, and you'll get varied recommendations from different people.

The best way to determine if a particular gemstone is good for you or for a specific chakra is to "test" it by placing it on your body and checking in with your body's subtle (or sometimes, not-so-subtle) response.

You may even want to have a friend place different stones on your body while your eyes are closed, so you can determine which ones genuinely feel the best on each chakra without being affected by your beliefs, or the way the rocks look.

Always trust your body's response. If a stone feels bad on your body, remove it, unless you recognize that "bad" feeling as a clearing, and feel an instinctive desire to stay with the stone.

Amethyst is a popular crown gemstone that reduces stress and expands spiritual awareness.

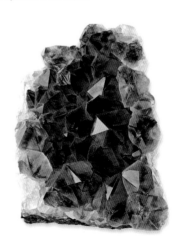

CHAKRA GEMSTONES ELEMENT MEDITATION

1. Choose seven stones—one for each chakra (see the lists on pages 160–163).

2. Lie down and place each stone on your body in its chakra location. The crown stone can go on the floor right above the head (like in the image below).

3. Close your eyes and soften into the rhythm of your breath. When you feel relaxed, focus on each stone and its element from the root upward:

ROOT—Imagine this stone comes from the core of the earth, stable and vital, and feel these grounded qualities in your tailbone, legs, and feet.

SACRAL—Imagine this stone comes from the bottom of the ocean, with the tides moving in and out of it, back and forth. Experience these easy, flowing energies in your pelvic bowl.

SOLAR PLEXUS—Imagine this stone comes from the center of the sun, infinitely bright and powerful, and feel these qualities living in your core.

HEART—Imagine this stone comes from the winds that blow, bringing renewal, peace, and love into your being. Feel your heart expand.

THROAT—Imagine this stone comes from the most soulful, moving music you've ever heard, reminding you of who you really are. Feel your authentic voice blossom in your throat.

BROW—Imagine this stone comes from the light of the universe, bringing clarity and strong intuition. Feel your third eye opening wider now.

CROWN—Imagine this stone comes straight from your Higher Power (or All That Is), bringing a sense of spiritual connection. Feel how you are one with absolutely everything.

4. If you have time, repeat the process moving back down your body, thanking each chakra and gemstone for bringing its gifts into your life.

5. When you're finished, open your eyes and put your seven healing stones on an altar, or somewhere you can see them as a reminder of balance.

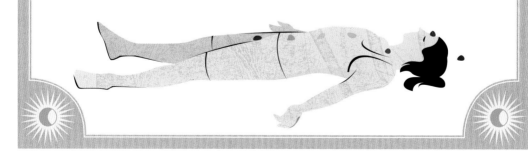

WORKING WITH COLORED STONES

A very simple but generally good rule for chakra balancing is that if a stone is the color of the chakra, it's good for boosting and balancing that chakra. Hence, the first chakra stones tend to be red-toned, the second chakra stones orange-toned, and so on.

Certain key stones—quartz, tourmaline, or calcite, for example—come in many different hues and can be used for all of the chakras, depending on their color.

A couple of the chakras have secondary colors that you should consider when picking gemstones. For the root chakra, the secondary color is black, and for the heart chakra it's pink.

This does not mean, though, that every stone that heals a particular chakra will be the primary or secondary color of that chakra. There are many exceptions. Still, there is so much correspondence between the gemstone colors and the chakras they balance that it is a great "rule of thumb"—especially for anyone who doesn't know a lot about rocks.

If you wish to experiment with some gemstones to see which ones feel right for you, here are some stones to consider for healing each chakra:

ROOT CHAKRA

- **Garnet**—promotes manifestation, revitalizes, releases guilt and inhibitions, purifies blood, and regenerates DNA
- **Ruby**—stimulates passion, determination, and prosperity; balances sex drive; detoxifies blood and lymph nodes
- **Hematite**—grounds, strengthens, and revitalizes; enhances memory; helps iron absorption and red blood cell creation
- **Red jasper**—promotes earth connection and stability, gently stimulates and protects, reduces worry and electromagnetic field pollution
- **Black tourmaline**—enhances goal manifestation; dispels stress and fear; treats bowels, colon, lower back, legs, and feet
- **Bloodstone**—grounds and helps one to face challenges, increases patience and ability to sacrifice, heals anemia

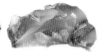

SACRAL CHAKRA

- **Orange carnelian**—increases passion, joy, creativity, motivation, and feminine energy; aids fertility and menses
- **Moonstone**—assists looking inward; calms and stabilizes emotions; helps PMS, fertility, childbirth, and breast-feeding
- **Coral**—enhances feminine fertility and passion, balances emotions, helps alleviate bladder issues
- **Fire opal**—accesses subconscious, releases attachment, fires up kundalini and joy, cures dehydration and water retention
- **Orange calcite**—lifts energy and spirit, clears emotional and reproductive issues, balances sexual energies
- **Amber**—promotes emotional ease, protects from energetic invasion, nurtures creativity, reduces stress, heals wounds

SOLAR PLEXUS CHAKRA

- **Citrine**—magnifies personal power, clarity and focus; helps alleviate fatigue
- **Topaz**—stimulates and recharges, clarifies intention, heals gout, and boosts appetite

- **Tiger's eye**—cultivates confidence, courage, and good judgment; benefits the pancreas
- **Fire agate**—increases courage, vigor, and willpower; helps to overcome addictions
- **Yellow apatite**—lifts energy, promotes optimism and self-confidence, enhances digestion
- **Golden calcite**—instills mental alertness and willpower; good for digestion and diaphragm

HEART CHAKRA

- **Aventurine**—increases good luck, encourages mature love, protects against pollutants, helps prevent heart attacks
- **Emerald (stone of Venus)**—fosters hope, preserves love, renews the spirit, wards off allergies
- **Jade**—promotes unconditional love and serenity, calms anger, boosts the immune system
- **Rose quartz**—helps foster forgiveness and self-love, strengthens the heart, heals respiratory issues
- **Pink tourmaline**—heals emotional wounds, boosts yin energy and love, helps angina and other heart issues
- **Moldavite**—activates the heart chakra, promotes wonder, heals asthma and allergies

THROAT CHAKRA

- **Aquamarine**—promotes heartfelt communication and courage; good for thyroid, sore throats, teeth, and gums
- **Blue calcite**—fosters enlightened conversations and learning, soothes and calms, heals tonsils and thyroid
- **Blue kyanite**—cleanses negative energy, improves communication and telepathy, good for parathyroid
- **Lapis lazuli**—fosters honor, truth, good judgment, and public success; benefits thyroid; helps with hearing loss
- **Sodalite**—helps heal breaches in communication, aids idealism and self-discipline, good for vocal chords
- **Turquoise**—promotes leadership, wisdom, and spiritual connection; detoxifies; cures speech disorders

BROW CHAKRA

- **Azurite**—opens the third eye; enhances dreams, balance, and new perspectives; soothes migraines; aids Alzheimer's
- **Barite**—promotes inner vision and dream recall, gently removes blocks, increases *chi*, balances brain chemistry
- **Blue iolite**—boosts imagination and clairvoyance, calms the mind for meditation, balances yin–yang energies
- **Fluorite**—promotes intuition, interdimensional communication, and clear unbiased reasoning
- **Purple charoite**—opens one to spiritual guidance, past life lessons, and being in the now; heals eye issues and headaches
- **Labradorite**—boosts spiritual energy, clears and protects the aura, helps with eye and brain disorders
- **Indigo kyanite**—stimulates the pineal gland, cleanses negativity and fatalism, purifies the body and lifts vibration

KEYNOTE

You can do more focused healing by using a crystal wand—buy one or make your own by gluing colored stones or other talismans onto a pointed quartz crystal. Use the pointed end to direct the energy toward a specific spot like a chakra or a painful area.

CROWN CHAKRA

- **Amethyst**—enhances inner peace, spiritual awareness, meditation, and innovation; reduces stress and insomnia
- **Violet sapphire**—promotes spiritual understanding, prosperity, and good judgment; regulates glands
- **Clear quartz**—amplifies energy, thought, and intention; aids concentration and memory; cures pains and dizziness
- **Opal**—boosts imagination, optimism, memory, and potential; breaks through spiritual obstacles; aids eyes; reduces fever
- **White calcite**—amplifies energy, healing, and wisdom; reduces stress; heals past life karma; detoxifies
- **Diamond**—promotes spiritual illumination, good ethics, pure faith, and alignment; purifies; combats aging

HOW TO INFUSE YOUR LIFE WITH GEMSTONE ENERGY

Wearing or holding stones are not the only way to take in their healing energy. You can invest in a big centerpiece stone, like an exquisite amethyst, and enjoy it as art. This will boost the energy of your home or office and give your eyes a feast as well.

Another great way to keep healing stone energy around you is to get a Himalayan salt lamp. Its color is a pleasing pink, and it boosts the heart chakra, as well as the third eye. Salt is hygroscopic, so it attracts water molecules from the surrounding air. A large block of Himalayan salt attracts pollutants, so they're no longer floating in the air where you can inhale them. When it heats up, it also releases negative ions that boost blood flow, improve sleep, increase levels of serotonin in the brain, and calm allergy or asthma symptoms.

Finally, my favorite way to take in crystal energy is to imbibe it. No, I don't eat the stones. I keep seven beautiful quartz crystals in my water dispenser, so that all the water I drink is infused with powerful quartz energy. I also think the crystals make the water taste fresher. Try it yourself!

HEALING THE CHAKRAS WITH COLOR AND FOOD

Many people underestimate the ability of color to heal the chakras. This could be due to the fact that it seems too simple. But the truth is, color is a huge aspect of chakra healing, and using it to balance them is not only effective, but fun.

There are three main ways you can use color to heal your chakras: look at it, wear it, or eat it. In other words, you can use more color awareness when you design the spaces you spend time in, or when you choose the clothes you wear and food you eat. In the previous section, we talked about the power of using or wearing colored gemstones for healing.

Here again are the colors of the chakras:

Root—red
Throat—blue
Sacral—orange
Brow—indigo
Solar plexus—yellow
Crown—violet/white
Heart—green

Typically, we're drawn to the colors that are associated with our most open chakras. When I had a chronically weak root chakra and a super-strong crown, my favorite color was purple and I avoided red.

Once you know what your most underactive chakra is, start cultivating an appreciation for that chakra's color. The simplest way is to buy some articles of clothing, and also some key household items in that hue.

If you're willing to make a bigger commitment, paint a room or buy some drapes or furniture in that color to create big frequency shifts. And if you have a nice yard or garden, plant some flowers or vegetables in the color of the chakra you most need to heal and embrace.

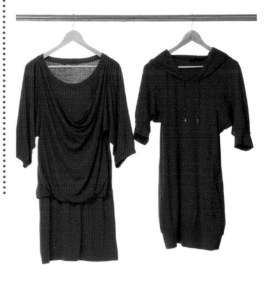

Wearing red not only helps you to stand out, but it grounds you and gives you vitality too.

CHAKRA HEALING FOODS

Perhaps one of the strongest ways you can incorporate chakra color into your life is through food, because you not only look at it, but you handle it, and consume it as well. This means it affects you from both the outside and the inside.

Each chakra has numerous foods that boost and balance it. Color is one of the biggest aspects of the healing, but there are other factors to consider as well. Things like the element and primary focus of the chakra play a big role. Also, every chakra is associated with a food type. When you take all of these factors into account, you can determine the most healing foods for each chakra.

One of the greatest things about using food for chakra healing is that it continually stimulates your chakra awareness. Since we have to eat every day, it invites us to stay mindful of our body's ongoing need for optimal energy and to consume the best foods we can to love and empower ourselves.

ROOT CHAKRA FOODS
Proteins and Meats

The red root chakra is about stability, and it's also related to proteins and the earth element. You can boost it by eating red, earthy, high-protein foods like beets, red meats, and red beans. And because fungi are also earthy, all edible mushrooms are good for the base chakra.

SACRAL CHAKRA FOODS
Liquids

The orange sacral chakra is associated with liquids and fluid foods, especially sensual ones. Fruit juices like mango, orange, and carrot really boost it. And foods with aphrodisiac qualities are good for it too, especially if they are fluid or come from the sea, like oysters.

Dark chocolate is another great aphrodisiac that boosts all of the feminine (even) chakras, because it releases the love hormone oxytocin (for the heart) and also boosts the brain, which is related to the third eye.

SOLAR PLEXUS CHAKRA FOODS
Carbohydrates

Because the solar plexus is associated with the fire element and with the stomach area, spicy foods really get it going. This is particularly true of gingerroot, because it's spicy with a light yellow hue and helps with indigestion.

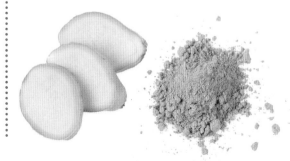

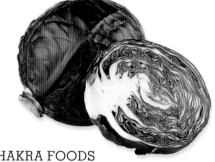

The solar plexus loves healthy carbohydrates because they can be quickly converted into energy, so most grains open the core. The color and versatility of corn make it a surefire bet. A spicy corn dish will really light up your solar plexus chakra!

HEART CHAKRA FOODS
Vegetables

The heart chakra is green and related to vegetables, so you have plenty to choose from such as green beans, all types of lettuce, peas, green bell peppers, zucchini, squash, and more. They are great fresh, but since the heart is the air chakra, you can also eat them dried.

THROAT CHAKRA FOODS
Fruits

Once we move into the upper chakras and the spiritual realm, there are far less food associations, since these chakras are more about your spiritual development than your body or its nourishment. Still, the throat chakra's food type is fruit and its Sanskrit name, visuddha, means "purity," so any foods that detoxify are good. The powerful antioxidant properties and color of blueberries make them the perfect food for healing the throat chakra. Thyroid-healing foods like sea plants, dandelion greens, turmeric, liver, scallops, and oysters are great too.

BROW CHAKRA FOODS
Presentation

To open the brow chakra (third eye), eat indigo or purplish foods such as grapes, blackberries, and "red" cabbage. Or dive into nourishment that has brain-boosting capacities such as coconut oil, eggs, walnuts, or dark chocolate. To open the brow chakra, make sure to present your meals in ways that please the eye!

CROWN CHAKRA FOODS
Fasting

Finally, the crown is connected to the spiritual realm, so it's about abstaining from the foods that feed our physical flesh. In this way, you can reduce your psychological dependence on food and also detoxify.

If you decide to fast, be sure you only do so for a responsible length of time, and drink lots of structured, high-alkaline water. I share a simple way to create structured quartz water on page 163.

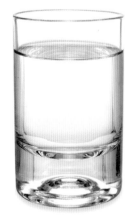

BEST CHAKRA FOODS AND SPICES

Root

- beets
- red meat
- red beans
- red potatoes
- strawberries
- cherries
- mushrooms
- Tazo's Passion Tea (it's bright red!)

Sacral

- orange juice
- carrot juice
- mangos
- passion fruit
- sweet potatoes or pumpkin (especially as soup)
- salmon
- oysters
- dark chocolate

Solar Plexus

- corn
- ginger
- potatoes
- spicy hummus
- papaya
- pineapple
- polenta
- couscous
- cayenne
- cumin
- turmeric
- yellow curry

Heart

- green beans
- green bell peppers
- kale and all types of lettuce
- peas
- cucumbers
- zucchini
- avocados
- alfalfa and bean sprouts
- lima beans
- wheatgrass
- celery
- asparagus
- Brussels sprouts
- parsley
- broccoli
- dark chocolate

Throat

- blueberries
- sea plants
- dandelion greens
- scallops
- turmeric
- liver
- oysters

Brow

- blackberries
- purple grapes
- red cabbage
- raisins
- prunes
- coconut oil
- eggs
- walnuts
- dark chocolate
- beautifully arranged foods

Crown

- fasting
- water (structured quartz, high alkaline)

HEALING THE CHAKRAS WITH MEDITATION

Guided meditation is a great way to explore and heal your chakras, because energy responds to intention instantaneously and meditation allows you to focus your intentions while in a very relaxed state. I have included several guided meditations in this book: see pages 19, 159, 169, and 182.

You can also create your own meditation. It's really easy. Simply close your eyes, set a healing intention, and go to the area of each chakra in your mind's eye. If you are feeling heavy or depressed and need inspiration, start at the root chakra and work your way up. Conversely, if you are feeling anxious or need grounding, begin at the crown and work your way down.

As you move up or down, visualize the color of each chakra, or imagine the animal, deity, archetype (or any other related symbol) for that chakra.

CHAKRA MEDITATION SYMBOLS

Here are some animals, deities, archetypes, and other symbols you can incorporate into your meditations:
- **Root**—elephant, tortoise, bear, Ganesha, tree, mountain, Mother Earth
- **Sacral**—pairs of dolphins, otters and water eels, Goddess Venus, belly dancer, ocean, moon
- **Solar plexus**—lion, ram, horse, dragon, Lord Rama, volcano, fire, sun

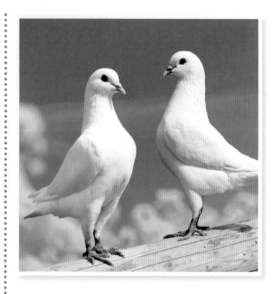

Doves are a great heart chakra symbol as they invoke both peace and love.

- **Heart**—doves (and other birds), antelope, deer, Tara, Quan Yin, Hanuman, heart symbol, cross
- **Throat**—blue-throated hummingbird, dragonfly, whale
- **Brow**—owl, eagle, crystal ball, eye, peacock
- **Crown**—butterfly, rainbow, Shiva, royal crown, angel

DAILY CHAKRA BALANCING MEDITATION

The most important chakra meditation of all is this basic one. Done consistently, it will help your energy fields stay strong, open, and balanced. A simple visualization meditation, it is perfect for boosting, balancing, and cleansing your chakras on a daily basis. If possible, record it, so you can listen to the replay with your eyes closed.

1. Find a comfortable, seated position and close your eyes.

2. Focus on your breath and feel into its natural rhythm, as it moves in and out. Notice how each inhale gently expands your chest, and each exhale allows you to release and relax. Inhale . . . expand . . . exhale . . . relax. Inhale . . . expand . . . exhale . . . relax.

3. Now, take your attention down to your tailbone. Here, imagine strong, red roots growing downward into the Earth's core. See or feel these roots wrapping themselves around the Earth's core, and as they do, feel how they make you more stable and grounded.

4. Inhale vital Earth energy from the core of the Earth up to the bottom of your heart and hold it for just a moment, then exhale it upward through your crown, like a whale's spout.

5. Imagine your crown opening wide like a funnel, and inhale Sky energy down through your crown into your heart, hold it just a moment, and exhale it down into Mother Earth.

6. Once again, inhale from the Earth's core up into your heart, and exhale up to the sky. Inhale from the sky down into your heart, exhale down into Mother Earth.

7. One more time, inhale up to your heart, exhale to the sky. Inhale down into your heart. Exhale into the Earth.

8. Place both of your hands on your heart center, one on top of the other, and thank Mother Earth and Father Sky for feeding your energy body.

9. Gently open your eyes and enjoy the calm, energized feeling of balanced chakras.

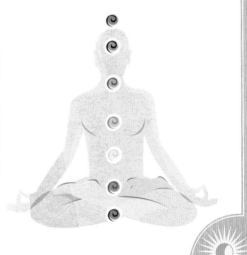

HEALING WITH YOUR HANDS

Your hands are great tools for healing because they are an extension of your heart chakra. And, each of your palms has a "minor" chakra in its center that, when activated, puts out healing energy. Unfortunately, at this point in time there are no well-known energy healing methods that directly address and incorporate the seven main chakras. But there is one modality that benefits your chakras and is fairly popular across the globe. It's called Reiki and it involves the "laying on of hands," either literally or remotely, to move life-force energy in a way that relaxes and heals the receiver.

The International Center for Reiki Training estimates there are over four million people worldwide who have undertaken some Reiki training, and the Center for Reiki Research lists over 70 American hospitals currently offering Reiki healings.

It seems that we are ushering in a new era where energy healing modalities are gradually being embraced by the medical community. If you'd like to do energy healing as a complement to allopathic or conventional medicine, consider learning Reiki. Many schools and teachers all over the world offer certification.

If you want to explore using your hands to directly balance the chakras, do my Open Heart Chakra Healing exercise (on the facing page). It shows you how to open your heart, connect with Source, and do a basic chakra healing. Try it out and see how it works for you. Feel free to modify it according to your own needs and intuition.

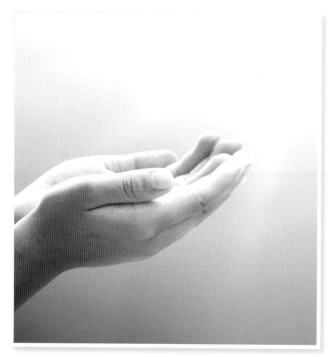

Your hands emit powerful, healing heart energy.

OPEN HEART CHAKRA HEALING PROCESS

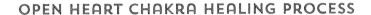

1. Have the person receiving the healing lie on their back on a massage table (or if one is not available, use a bed).

2. While gazing at the person receiving the healing, lightly touch the middle of your chest with the fingers of your dominant hand to establish a heart connection with them.

3. Keeping that, open your other hand out to the side with your palm facing up to establish a connection with the Divine.

4. In this position, say a little prayer to yourself to call in assistance from the Divine Source of your choosing. If you like, you can use this one: "Universe (or your Source Name), please use me as an instrument of Divine Healing for this beautiful being before me. Amen."

5. Open your hand chakras by lifting both arms in front of you with one palm up and one palm down. Open and close your fists quickly about a dozen times and then flip your hands and repeat.

6. Stand on one side of the table by their head with your elbows bent. Align your dominant hand slightly above your non-dominant hand and hold both above the receiver's crown chakra area (at a height that is comfortable for you).

7. Make at least seven small (saucer-size) clockwise circles with your hands. You may notice tingling or a slight taffy-like pull.

8. Do the same for the rest of the chakras, moving down the body from the third eye to the root chakra. If any intuitive images or ideas arise, you can ask the person you are healing if they would like you to share them. Sometimes divine messages come through the healer.

9. After you've done the root, place your hands on the receiver's ankles and give them a gentle squeeze to ground them back into their body and signal the end of the healing.

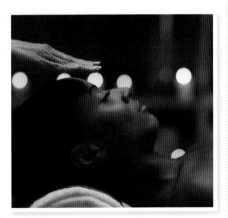

While focusing on each chakra, you can use one hand, as shown here, or two hands (described above).

EMOTIONAL FREEDOM TECHNIQUE (AKA TAPPING)

Emotional Freedom Technique, popularly known as EFT or Tapping, was created by Dr. Roger Callahan in the early 1980s and then refined by Stanford engineer Gary Craig in the early 1990s. Basically, EFT is an emotional version of acupuncture without the needles. It invites you to bring up an emotional issue and then tap on your key meridian points until the energy shifts and your nervous system calms down. Based on a Chinese healing system that has been used effectively for thousands of years, EFT has been proven effective by numerous scientific studies over the last two decades.

Since many chakra blockages begin in the emotional energy body, EFT can be a powerful way to break through emotional stuck points and open up your energy field without rehashing emotional memories or paying for many years of therapy.

You can't go wrong with EFT. It's one of the easiest, quickest healing processes and the internet is full of great EFT videos and other resources to guide you through this simple process. So the next time you feel any sticky chakra issues, just tap them out!

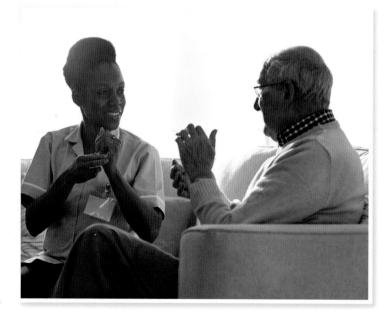

↓ Tapping is easy to learn and has been proven to effectively reduce stress in numerous studies.

HOW TO PERFORM EFT

In order to perform EFT, first memorize the Nine Basic Tapping Points in the illustration below, then follow these steps.

1. Identify the issue you want to address in a clear and simple way. For example, we'll address the root chakra issue of being bad with money.

2. Measure the intensity of your issue with a baseline measurement so you can see if it improves after EFT. Rate the issue on a scale of 0 to 10 where 10 means the issue is the worst it could ever be, and 0 means it's not a problem at all.

3. Create a simple issue statement. Be blunt and don't try to soften it. You actually want your body to have its typical, negative reaction so you can tap on it and neutralize it. Use this statement template:

Even though I have (or I am) _____, I accept and love myself completely.

In our example, it would be, *"Even though I'm bad with money, I accept and love myself completely."*

4. Say your statement repeatedly as you tap through the EFT points with the tips of two or three fingers of your dominant hand. Start at the top of the head and make your way down to the karate chop point, tapping roughly five to seven times at each point.

5. After you've gone through all the points once or twice, stop and rate the intensity of the issue. If it's gone down enough for your satisfaction, you are done.

6. If you feel you haven't reduced the intensity level enough, repeat steps 4 and 5 until you get the results you want.

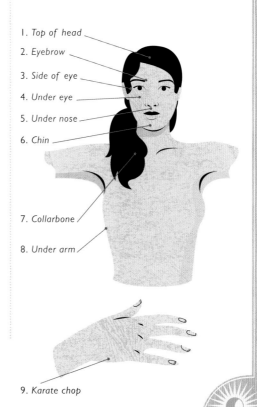

1. *Top of head*
2. *Eyebrow*
3. *Side of eye*
4. *Under eye*
5. *Under nose*
6. *Chin*
7. *Collarbone*
8. *Under arm*
9. *Karate chop*

TRANSFORMATIONAL POWER QUESTIONS (TPQS)

Over the last few decades, affirmations have become a popular healing tool for personal growth, because they're easy to do and they seem so good for you. But the truth is, for many people, especially those who lack a strong solar plexus chakra, affirmations can do more harm than good. This is why I like to use a variation on traditional affirmations that I call Transformational Power Questions (TPQs). They work great for everybody and they are easy to do.

Before I show you how to create effective TPQs, let me explain why affirmations can sometimes have a negative, rather than positive, effect.

Your most powerful and prominent mind is not your conscious mind, but your subconscious. It more or less runs your life. When you say a positive affirmation like "I am rich," that you don't believe is true, your subconscious tends to negate it with comments like "No you're not," or "Who are you kidding? You can't even pay your bills!" So for every one positive affirmation you say, you may get numerous negative rebuttals.

Try it yourself right now. Think of something big you'd like to have in your life that feels out of reach and turn it into a simple affirmation. Or just use this one: "I am famous." Say it and then be quiet and notice how your subconscious responds. If you can't hear or feel any resistance, direct affirmations may work great for you.

But if you can feel or hear resistance to the affirmation, then you will likely have much better luck using TPQs, because they engage your powerful subconscious mind in a positive way, and make it work for you, not against you. Create some and see for yourself!

HOW TO CREATE TPQS

Here's what you do to create a TPQ:

1. Think of something you want to change (i.e., be more patient)
2. Write a simple affirmation: *"I am patient."*
3. Turn it into a Why question: *"Why am I so patient?"*
4. Make it progressive: *"Why am I becoming more patient every day?"*

Ask your TPQ several times throughout the day. It's best to focus on one for a little while until you feel a shift, and then start on another.

Here are two good TPQs for each chakra to get you started:

Here are two good TPQs for each chakra to get you started:

ROOT CHAKRA TPQS

- Why am I becoming more abundant every day?
- Why am I becoming continually more stable and grounded?

SACRAL CHAKRA TPQS

- Why am I getting sexier every day?
- Why am I becoming continually more comfortable with my emotions?

SOLAR PLEXUS CHAKRA TPQS

- Why am I allowing myself to enjoy more and more success?
- Why am I growing more confident every day?

HEART CHAKRA TPQS

- Why am I experiencing more and more love in my life?
- Why am I more forgiving to myself and others every day?

THROAT CHAKRA TPQS

- Why am I continually becoming my most authentic self?
- Why am I stepping into my highest purpose more every day?

BROW CHAKRA TPQS

- Why is my third eye continually opening?
- Why are my intuition and psychic skills growing stronger every day?

CROWN CHAKRA TPQS

- Why is my connection to the Divine continually growing?
- Why is my spiritual wisdom and faith expanding every day?

Notice how these "why" questions invite your subconscious mind to respond with lots of good reasons why the TPQ is true. It's really powerful! So why not create some of your own and turbo-boost your personal expansion?

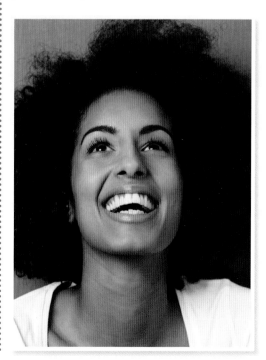

TPQs empower you by shifting your subconscious beliefs.

THE BEST HEALING METHODS FOR EACH CHAKRA

Now that we've gone over many effective chakra healing modalities, you're probably wondering which one is best. The definitive answer is, *it depends*. Each chakra is totally unlike the others, so the best method differs depending on which chakra you want to heal. Most of the modalities I've shared are good for balancing *all* of your chakras. Still, if you want to heal one particular chakra, it's best to choose the ideal techniques for that specific energy center.

My Chakra Boosters Healing Tattoos™ are perfect for addressing individual chakras. I created them after discovering the work of Dr. Masaru Emoto, which shows that symbols positively affect the molecular structure of water. I suddenly realized that since humans are mostly water, putting a Sanskrit root symbol right on my tailbone could possibly heal my first chakra. And that's exactly what happened. The moment the tattoo artist put the stencil of the root chakra design on my tailbone, a surge of energy rushed down my legs into the earth and I was instantly grounded! From that moment on, I knew I *had* to create temporary chakra tattoos so others could experience the same kind of healing.

CHAKRA MODALITIES

Chakra	Sense	Element
Root	Smell	Earth
Sacral	Taste	Water
Solar Plexus	Sight	Fire
Heart	Touch	Air
Throat	Hearing	Sound
Brow	"Sixth" sense	Light
Crown	None	Consciousness

One way to determine which healing methods are best is to look at the bodily sense and natural element for the chakra you want to heal and find the modalities that encompass them. These are shown in the table on the facing page.

BEST HEALING METHODS FOR YOUR ROOT CHAKRA

 Your root chakra is related to your sense of smell, so aromatherapy works wonders here. Use earthy, woodsy, or musky scents. Some of the aromatherapy oils for your first chakra are cedarwood, black spruce, patchouli, rosewood, sandalwood, and vetiver (see pages 126 and 129).

Since your root chakra is all about embodiment, the best, long-term healing comes from very physical activities like Hatha yoga, especially if you practice the second Principle of Alignment, Muscular Contraction, and do strong standing or squatting poses. And since your feet are ground zero for your base chakra, getting a reflexology treatment, or even just a good foot massage, is powerful root medicine.

You can also use earthy gemstones and crystals, especially the red and black ones like garnet, ruby, hematite, and black tourmaline. Gardening, hiking, and communing with trees are all great root-boosting activities, because they connect you to Mother Earth.

Playing or listening to indigenous music boosts the first chakra. Drumming to a tribal beat is powerful, as is listening to the didgeridoo, an Aboriginal instrument that vibrates with low, earthy tones.

Finally, you can wear my root Chakra Boosters Healing Tattoo™ at the lowest part of your back, near your tailbone. For super grounding, you can also wear two extra root tattoos, one at the top of each thigh.

KEYNOTE

For a really unique way to boost your root chakra with aromas, simply recreate your favorite smells from childhood. This will impart a deep sense of home and belonging, and it may flood you with sweet memories too.

BEST HEALING METHODS FOR YOUR SACRAL CHAKRA

 Your sacral chakra is all about your emotions, pleasure, sexuality, surrender, and joy, so look for modalities and activities that open up any of these areas and relate to your sense of taste and the element of water.

Tantric exercises or other forms of sacred sexuality work really well, as does yoga, especially if you focus on doing vinyasa flow, hip-opening poses, and the third Principle of Alignment, Inner Spiral, which is described on page 155.

A really good sensual Swedish-style massage will expand your sacral chakra, and a juice fast with fresh squeezed orange fruits such as mangos or oranges will too.

Since your sacral chakra is your feelings center, emotional release techniques are healing. A few effective ones you can look into are Heart IQ, NLP's Emotional Release Technique, and Emotional Freedom Technique, which is described on page 173.

Dancing is really good for the sacral chakra, especially the hip-swiveling types of movement like Zumba, Salsa, and belly dancing.

Any kind of aquatic therapy heals the second chakra. One of the best techniques is Watsu, the practice of being gently held and guided in water. It invites you to surrender completely to the healer, and letting go is the essence of this chakra.

You can also wear my sacral Chakra Boosters Healing Tattoo™ under your navel, or between your sacral divots on your lower back. If you have past sexual or emotional trauma, begin with the back (as that literally represents the past) and then add the front when you are feeling stronger.

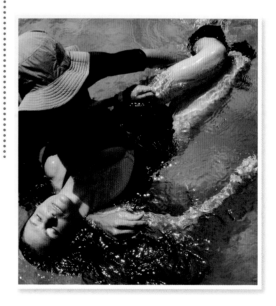

♀ Watsu, an aquatic form of body work, is the quintessential sacral chakra healing technique.

BEST HEALING METHODS FOR YOUR SOLAR PLEXUS CHAKRA

Since your solar plexus chakra is the fire element and is related to your sense of sight, gazing steadily at a burning flame or fiery yantra (a symmetrical yogic symbol) quickly strengthens it.

The solar plexus is the center of the conscious, thinking mind, so doing puzzles and brain teasers boosts its energy. Sunbathing is good too, especially done in a meditative way, where you imagine you are literally absorbing the sun's power.

Any method that builds confidence boosts third chakra energy. One great technique is to ask Transformational Power Questions (TPQs), see page 174.

Physically working on your core with Pilates or any core-oriented type of yoga is great for your solar plexus chakra. And taking any kind of courageous action, like fire-walking, boosts it as well.

Wearing my third Chakra Boosters Healing Tattoo™ on your solar plexus will also immediately give you a boost of confidence and "can do." If you have self-esteem issues that stem from the past, wear one on your back for a while before wearing one on the front, so your courage and confidence come from authenticity, rather than bravado.

One breathing exercise that many yogis do to boost their solar plexus chakra is *"breath of fire."* If you do it regularly, you'll build a strong and powerful core.

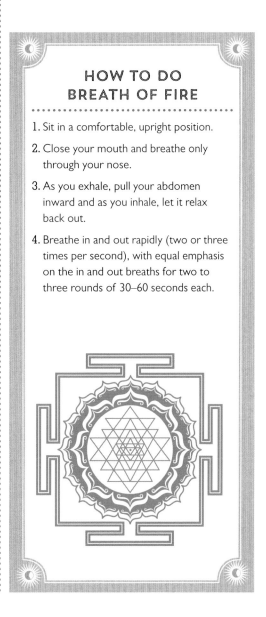

HOW TO DO BREATH OF FIRE

1. Sit in a comfortable, upright position.
2. Close your mouth and breathe only through your nose.
3. As you exhale, pull your abdomen inward and as you inhale, let it relax back out.
4. Breathe in and out rapidly (two or three times per second), with equal emphasis on the in and out breaths for two to three rounds of 30–60 seconds each.

BEST HEALING METHODS FOR YOUR HEART CHAKRA

 Because the heart chakra is related to your sense of touch, hugging is probably its most powerful healing technique. Our culture vastly underestimates the therapeutic value of a good hug.

Studies show that babies thrive when nurses and nannies hold them, and adults do too. Hugging is one of the simplest ways to boost and balance the heart chakra, so share as many hugs as you can every day.

Emotional Freedom Technique (EFT) is also great for the heart chakra, because it's about literally touching (tapping on) the body (page 173 describes how to perform it). And as you might imagine, all forms of breath work heal the heart chakra, because the element is air and our lungs connect to our heart. Set the intention to breath more deeply every day.

Since your heart chakra energy moves down your arms and is naturally expressed through your hands, you can boost it with any hand-oriented, energy healing techniques like Reiki or the Open Heart Chakra Healing Process on page 171.

One of the best ways to expand your heart chakra is to genuinely forgive both yourself and others. My favorite technique for this is the Hawaiian forgiveness practice known as Ho'Oponopono. I offer a popular, guided Ho'Oponopono meditation on YouTube.

You can also open your heart chakra by wearing my fourth Chakra Boosters Healing Tattoo™ on the center of your chest or between your shoulder blades. Wearing the tattoo on your back will help you grieve and heal any heart losses and wearing it on the front will help you express more love as you move forward in your life.

When we hug, our body releases oxytocin that lowers our heart rate and blood pressure.

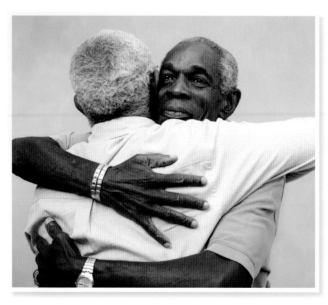

BEST HEALING METHOD FOR YOUR THROAT CHAKRA

 One highly effective way to open your fifth chakra is sound healing. Try playing a pure crystal bowl or tuning fork that is designed for opening the throat. Or you can simply listen to music or sounds that make you happy, calm, and centered.

It's also good to chant Sanskrit (yoga-related) mantras. My favorite mantra for the throat is "Om shree Vaka, jaya Vaka," which I use in the chorus of my throat chakra song on my healing album, *Chakra Love.*

Because the throat is the perfect place for a necklace and it's a masculine chakra like the root, you may want to wear a strong, fifth chakra stone pendant, like turquoise or lapis lazuli, around your neck.

If you have a serious throat chakra imbalance, doing shoulder stands helps immensely. It stimulates the thyroid gland that keeps your fifth chakra balanced. A good friend of mine alleviated all symptoms of Graves' disease by doing one 3-minute headstand followed by one 3-minute shoulder stand every day for six months.

My throat Chakra Boosters Healing Tattoo™ is another powerful way to open your throat and get in touch with your authentic voice. Wear it on the back of your neck.

VOCAL EXERCISE TO OPEN YOUR THROAT CHAKRA

1. Find a place where you feel comfortable being loud, and won't be disturbed.

2. Sitting cross-legged or in a chair, open your arms wide to the sky and yell "YES!" then wrap your arms around your chest as if you're hugging yourself and bow your head forward as you yell "NO!"

3. Alternate back and forth yelling "YES!" and "NO!"

You may find that it's easier to do one than the other. Keep practicing until you can say both words equally loud and strong.

BEST HEALING METHODS FOR YOUR BROW CHAKRA

 Active meditations are great for opening the third eye and they're easy to do. You simply close your eyes and purposely create a positive world within. Try the elevator meditation described in the panel here.

Visualizing and making a vision board boosts the brow chakra too. I offer a free video series on my Chakra Boosters YouTube channel that guides you through a soulful vision board process, but you can easily make one on your own. Simply buy a large foam core board and start pasting images on it that passionately inspire you in every area of your life!

Of course, you can also boost your third eye by wearing my brow Chakra Boosters Healing Tattoo™ while you sleep. You don't have to "wear" it. Just place it on your forehead, sticky side down, before bed and take it off in the morning. This way, you get the energetic benefit, without having people stare at your forehead!

ELEVATOR MEDITATION FOR OPENING YOUR THIRD EYE

1. Find a comfortable seated position, close your eyes, and relax.

2. Imagine your spine is an elevator shaft and each chakra is a different floor. Currently, your elevator is stopped at the third eye "floor."

3. Ask your elevator to come to the floor you're operating from now. Intuitively, it will go to one of your chakras.

4. When it arrives, imagine a miniature you stepping into the elevator and being carried all the way up to the third eye.

5. Step out of the elevator and look out the "window" of your brow chakra. From this vast perspective, ask your Higher Self any question, and an answer will intuitively come. When you've asked enough, thank your Higher Self, and gently open your eyes.

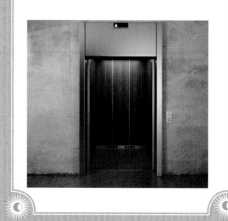

BEST HEALING METHODS FOR THE CROWN CHAKRA

For the seventh chakra, practicing meditation is best. The purer and simpler it is, the better. Gently close your eyes, watch your breath, and be a silent witness to your own mind and body. Don't try to change anything. Just notice it all: how your body feels and what emotions or thoughts are coming up. If you have a judgment about anything that pops up, just witnessing it in a nonjudgmental way will expand your seventh chakra.

Praying or communicating in any way with your Higher Power is a great way to open your crown chakra. If you have an angel guide or loved one who has passed, communicating with them will help open your crown as well.

Fasting boosts your crown too. Because we eat to feed the body and our seventh chakra is above the body, fasting naturally opens our spiritual awareness. If you can get past the hunger pangs and the discomfort, you can free up energy that would normally be mentally and physically preoccupied with food.

Wearing my crown Chakra Booster Healing Tattoo™ is good too. But since not all of us can wear it on the top of our head, it's best to place it on your "high heart"—on your back between your neck and shoulder blades.

QUICK CROWN CHAKRA-OPENING VISUALIZATION

1. Sit upright comfortably and close your eyes.

2. Observe the way your breath moves, and gently encourage it to deepen and slow down.

3. When you feel relaxed, imagine you have a sunroof at the top of your head.

4. Pretend that you are pushing a button and envision this sunroof slowly opening.

5. As it opens, imagine warm golden light filling you up. Feel it's healing your every cell.

6. When you feel completely filled with warm energy, gently open your eyes.

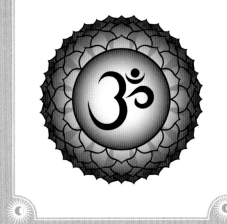

THE FUTURE OF CHAKRA HEALING

As our collective consciousness expands on this planet, more and more people are becoming aware of the fact that we are spiritual beings made of energy and that our chakras are a template for healing issues in many areas of our lives. This is a great advancement, but I think we need to take our perspective further and see that the chakras are more than just a vehicle for healing and problem solving. They're a map for developing new capacities, and for creating planetary peace and wellness.

GOING BEYOND HEALING

We don't need anything to be going wrong in our lives for us to work with our energy centers. We're at a key turning point in our collective evolution where we can live in an expanded way.

Perhaps there's a good reason why we have long been captivated by myths of gods and goddesses, or in more recent times, by superheroes. Our fascination with "supernatural" abilities may just be reflecting our own inner knowing that our potential is much greater than we have realized so far.

What if "supernatural" abilities are just that—extremely natural? What if telepathy, clairvoyance, and skills like levitation are just natural, expanded ways of being?

I know that personally, ever since I began healing my chakra "issues," my intuitive and empathic abilities as well as my health have continued to expand.

And it feels like this is only the beginning; like the sky is the limit.

We all can and should continue to work with our chakras even when we don't have any symptoms, problems, or needs. We should make discovering and living our highest potential our greatest aim.

UNDERSTANDING OUR ENERGETIC LIFE CYCLES

In the fall of 2012, something very exciting happened—I "downloaded" a year-by-year blueprint for human spiritual evolution that's tied to our chakras. Suddenly, I knew the reason why infants go through their "terrible twos," why so many relationships experience a "seven-year itch," why midlife crises happen, and so much more!

I call this blueprint the Chakra Life Cycle System® (CLCS), and I've used it to help my clients navigate their lives with more self-love, courage, and acceptance.

As a race, we have long understood our biological developmental cycles, and this has enabled us to move through difficult, physical stages (like puberty and menopause) with grace. It's time for us to have the same understanding of our energetic evolution, so we can weather our challenging spiritual transitions with clarity and faith.

The Chakra Life Cycle System® shows how we develop a new chakra every seven years, starting with our root chakra from womb to age seven, sacral chakra from age eight to 14, solar plexus chakra from age 15 to 21, and so on. The CLCS also outlines our minor chakra life cycles that take place every year. I love teaching the CLCS to my clients, because understanding these natural cycles helps everyone better facilitate their own spiritual development.

The same is true for all the tools and techniques shared in this book. I hope you will take the ones you like the most and make them part of your everyday life. Spiritual growth does not occur by accident, but by reverent intention and design. If we all do chakra work on a regular basis, not only will we expand our awareness as individuals, but together, we will co-create a higher collective consciousness and a healthier, happier, and more harmonious world.

Your chakras can do more than heal you, they can unlock your supernatural abilities and full potential.

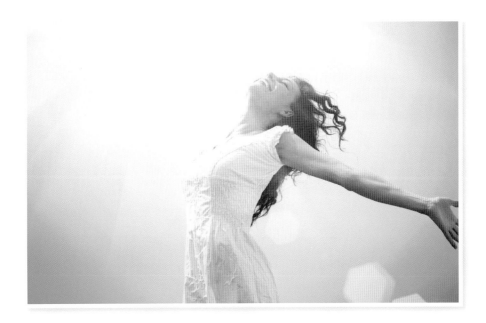

GLOSSARY

Applied kinesiology
A method of diagnosing energetic weakness and underlying illness by testing a subject's muscle strength.

Basic chakra needs
Seven human needs that relate to each chakra and develop early in life: the need for safety, variety, significance, love, true expression, intuitive connection, and oneness with the Divine.

Chakra life cycle system
A map of human energetic development that outlines the major and minor chakra energies that predominate every year of human life.

Chakra nexus point
The key balancing point directly between two adjacent chakras.

Emotional freedom technique (EFT)
A form of emotional healing that entails tapping on key acupressure points to restore energetic balance.

Endocrine system
The body's ductless glands that secrete key hormones that regulate the body, and interact with the chakras.

Grounding
Actually or meditatively connecting to Earth for more stability and security.

Healing crisis
Symptoms that arise after a healing process that indicate the body is creating a new energetic set point.

Ho'Oponopono
A meditative, Hawaiian method of love and forgiveness that heals the heart chakra.

Mantra
A repeated word or sound that aids concentration and healing.

Nadis
Energy currents of the subtle body.

Shiva/Shakti
The masculine/feminine Hindu deity with Shiva representing consciousness and Shakti representing form.

Transformational power questions (TPQs)
A healing method of turning traditional affirmations into "why" questions to positively engage the subconscious mind. An affirmation like "I am rich" becomes "Why am I getting wealthier every day?"

Yogic principles of alignment
A series of seven subtle movements (one for each chakra) that allow yoga practitioners to directly access and affect each chakra.

FURTHER READING

BOOKS

Dale, Cyndi.
Llewellyn's Complete Book of Chakras:
Your Definitive Source of Energy Center
Knowledge for Health, Happiness, and
Spiritual Evolution.
Woodbury, US, Llewellyn, 2016.

Judith, Anodea.
Anodea Judith's Chakra Yoga.
Woodbury, US, Llewellyn, 2015.

Judith, Anodea.
Wheels of Life: A User's Guide to the
Chakra System.
Woodbury, US, Llewellyn, 1987.

Goldman, Jonathan and Andi Goldman.
Chakra Frequencies: Tantra of Sound.
New York, US, Destiny Books, 2011.

Wauters, Ambika.
The Book of Chakras: Discover the
Hidden Forces Within You.
London, UK, Quarto, 2002.

USEFUL WEBSITES

Anusara Yoga
www.anusarayoga.com

Chakra Abundance
www.chakraabundance.com

Chakra Boosters
www.chakraboosters.com

Chakra Boosters Youtube Channel
www.youtube.com/chakraboosters

Eclectic Energies (chakra test)
www.eclecticenergies.com

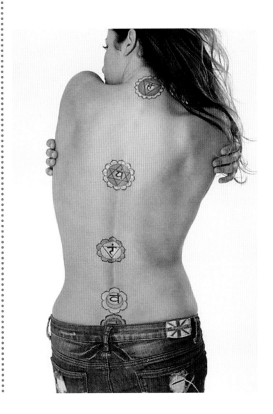

INDEX

CREDITS

∙∙

8 © wavebreakmedia | Shutterstock • 9, 33 © Nikki Zalewski | Shutterstock • 13 © Official | Shutterstock • 14 © Emilio Pastor de Miguel | Shutterstock • 15 © Jubair1985 | Creative Commons • 17 © Evgenia Kostiaeva | Shutterstock • 18 © Science Photo Library | Getty Images • 19, 161 right and middle left © vvoe | Shutterstock • 23 © andreiuc88 | Shutterstock • 25 © oorka | Shutterstock • 27 © Lukas Gojda | Shutterstock • 29 © Pazargic Liviu | Shutterstock • 31 © Billion Photos | Shutterstock • 35 © Klagyivik Viktor | Shutterstock • 38 © tantrik71 | Shutterstock • 39 © Winai Tepsuttinun | Shutterstock • 43 left © AWesleyFloyd| Shutterstock, right © Mad Dog | Shutterstock • 48 © Ljupco Smokovski | Shutterstock • 50 © Inneractive Enterprises, Inc. • 51 © OnlyZoia | Shutterstock • 51 © DeoSum | Shutterstock • 62 © Syda Productions | Shutterstock • 63 © zhu difeng | Shutterstock • 65 © Romolo Tavani | Shutterstock • 66 © Pikoso.kz | Shutterstock • 68 © Gts | Shutterstock • 69 © Chones | Shutetrstock • 70, 171 © Dragon Images | Shutterstock • 73 © Alena Ozerova | Shutterstock • 74 © Martin Novak | Shutterstock • 75 © Zurijeta | Shutterstock • 76 © paulaphoto | Shutterstock • 77 © sutipond | Shutterstock • 78 © Hulton Archive / Stringer | Getty Images • 79 © Baron / Stringer | Getty Images • 80 © Scott Legato / Stringer | Getty Images • 81 © Princess Diana Archive / Stringer | Getty Images • 82 © neftali | Shutterstock • 84 © baranq | Shutterstock • 94 © Monika Wisniewska | Shutterstock • 99 © jkerrigan | Shutterstock • 100 © Africa Rising | Shutterstock • 103 © Phase4Studios | Shutterstock • 105 © leungchopan | Shutterstock • 106 © Marcos Mesa Sam Wordley | Shutterstock • 107 © JPC-PROD | Shutterstock • 110 © igorstevanovic | Shutterstock • 111 © bikeriderlondon | Shutterstock • 113 © Lisa A | Shutterstock • 114 © pp1 | Shutterstock • 115 © aastock | Shutterstock • 120 © lzf | Shutterstock • 122 © Nadino | Shutterstock • 124 © Marie C Fields | Shutterstock • 125 © Botamochy | Shutterstock •126 left © marilyn barbone | Shutterstock, right © Anton-Burakov | Shutterstock • 127 top, 128 top right © Dionisvera | Shutterstock, bottom © JIANG HONGYAN | Shutterstock • 128 left © jopelka | Shutterstock, middle © azure1 | Shutterstock, right, 160 middle, 161 bottom right © Ilizia | Shutterstock, top left, 129 left © Scisetti Alfio | Shutterstock • 129 right © Irina Zavyalova | Shutterstock, top © Nik Merkulov | Shutterstock • 130 © Antonova Anna | Shutterstock • 131 © picturepartners | Shutterstock • 132 left © Anna Ok | Shutterstock, right © Copacabana | Shutterstock • 133 © Kotkoa | Shutterstock •134, 135, 179 © tschitscherin | Shutterstock • 135 bottom © Luis Molinero | Shutterstock • 136 © Zsolt Biczo | Shutterstock • 137 © Iakov Kalinin | Shutterstock • 138 © Ansis Klucis | Shutterstock • 139 © Axenova Alena | Shutterstock • 145 © The Cosmopolitan of Las Vegas | Creative Commons • 155 © nanka | Shutterstock • 156 © Surrphoto | Shutterstock • 157 © Mladen Mitrinovic | Shutterstock • 158 © Sebastian Janicki | Shutterstock • 160 left, 161 4th from left © Stellar Gems | Shutterstock, right, 161 middle right, 162 left © Imfoto | Shutterstock • 161 top left © MaraZe | Shutterstock, middle © J. Palys | Shutterstock, middle center © Byjeng | Shutterstock, bottom right © Chattranusorn09 | Shutterstock, bottom center, 162 2nd from left © Sergey Lavrentev | Shutterstock • 162 from left © Only Fabrizio | Shutterstock, © Martina Osmy | Shutterstock, © Albert Russ | Shutterstock • 163 left © J. Palys | Shutterstock, middle © J. Palys | Shutterstock, right © Beautyimage | Shutterstock • 164 top © NBeauty \ Shutterstock, bottom © 101imges | Shutterstock • 165 top © artintowninstock | Shutterstock, bottom © Viktor1 | Shutterstock • 166 top © Viktar Malyshchyts | Shutterstock, middle © COLOA Studio | Shutterstock, bottom © tanuha2001 | Shutterstock • 167 top left © Ildi Papp | Shutterstock, top right © KITSANANAN | Shutterstock, bottom left © Roman Tsubin | Shutterstock, bottom right © Yasonya | Shutterstock • 168 © Daniel Prudek | Shutterstock • 170 © CHOATphotographer | Shutterstock • 172 © Dean Mitchell | Getty Images • 175 © ESB Professional | Shuttertock • 178 © Dewi Putra | Shutterstock • 180 © Diego Cervo | Shutterstock • 187 © Shandon Youngclaus